THE LOVE DIET

THE LOVE DIET

A Personalized, Proven Program
That Changes the Way You Feel to
Transform the Way You Look

Connie Guttersen, R.D., Ph.D.
Mark Dedomenico, M.D.

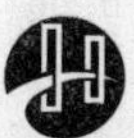

HarperOne
An Imprint of HarperCollins*Publishers*

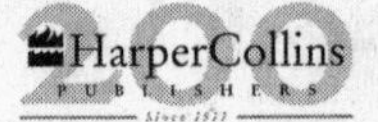

The Seven Stages plan found in *The Love Diet* has been used to treat many patients with obesity and metabolic disorders as well as other serious physical ailments. While almost anyone can engage in our plan, it is important to discuss this plan with your own doctor to confirm that it will present no risk to you personally. Your doctor's medical advice regarding the Seven Stages is particularly important if you're currently taking medications for diabetes, high cholesterol, high blood pressure, or any other metabolic disorders. Your doctor may need to adjust these medications as you progress through the program.

HarperCollins books may be purchased for educational, business, or sales promotional use. For information please e-mail the Special Markets Department at SPsales@harpercollins.com.

HarperCollins website: http://www.harpercollins.com

FIRST HARPERCOLLINS PAPERBACK EDITION PUBLISHED IN 2017

Designed by Joan Olson

Library of Congress Cataloging-in-Publication Data is available upon request.

ISBN 978-0-06-230304-2

17 18 19 20 21 LSC(H) 10 9 8 7 6 5 4 3 2 1

This book is dedicated to those who have decided to be healthier and happier.

When health is absent,
Wisdom cannot reveal itself,
Art cannot become manifest,
Strength cannot fight,
Wealth becomes useless,
And intelligence cannot be applied.

—Herophilus, Greek physician
(335–280 BCE)

Contents

Introduction

By Connie Guttersen, R.D., Ph.D.

Standing in line at the grocery store, you're likely to come face-to-face with magazine headlines touting competing "secrets" to diet success:

Eat fat to lose weight.

Carbs are the answer to long-term weight loss.

Fasting is the solution to drop unwanted pounds for good.

And magazines are only the tip of the iceberg. Health-centered TV shows and websites generate alleged weight loss solutions at an even faster clip. Even gatherings with friends and family aren't safe from influence—there seems to be an evangelist of the latest diet trend at every table.

Yet, despite the seemingly endless supply of information, nutritional clarity is at an all-time low. You're not alone if your head is spinning with conflicting dietary advice, or if you find it difficult to track down the most reliable information on how to eat best for health.

The result is a full-blown crisis of confidence. You've likely lost confidence in fad diet promises, so-called diet gurus, and—worst of all—yourself. Do you blame yourself for failing with diets? You shouldn't. It's not your fault.

When you're confused, you can't always figure out the right way to go. When you don't know what to eat, you're likely to head down the wrong path. When you follow a diet that doesn't work, the problems don't end when you've eaten your last bowl of cabbage soup or added butter to your morning coffee; in fact, they're just beginning. Unsuccessful dieting drops you into a cycle that is both emotionally and physically self-defeating. Emotionally, you enter into a space where the shame and guilt you feel over failure are all consuming. Physically, your body shifts into chemical imbalance. And where does this leave you? Well, with a loss of confidence in yourself and the dieting system.

There are major problems in the system that produces diets for public use: first, as already pointed out, most diets are often in conflict with one another; second, the credentials of many so-called diet experts are questionable, as are the less-than-clinical foundations of their programs; and third, the majority of diets have not been rigorously tested on significant numbers of the general population—people like you. These are some major weaknesses. But what if I told you that none of these issues touch on the core problem of most diets? What if I told you that there is another fundamental element missing that prevents you from achieving sustained weight loss?

You may have trouble believing this, but what is missing from all of these diet programs you've tried is self-respect and self-love. That's right: learning to love yourself is the key to experiencing freedom from the frustrating cycle of shame, guilt, and repeated weight gain.

This isn't just some feel-good mumbo jumbo; it's a golden truth proven through work with more than eleven thousand people. It's a truth that I discovered in my work with Dr. Mark Dedomenico, a pioneer in cardiovascular surgery and the acclaimed founder of the 20/20 LifeStyles program and the coauthor of this book. Through our extensive clinical research, we have found that self-acceptance, self-respect, and self-love are essential to successful and permanent weight loss.

It's well established that people with weight issues can develop a negative self-image. They often tell themselves things like "I can't stand myself," "I'm disgusting," "I'm a total failure," "I don't want to be seen in public," "I can't maintain a normal weight" . . . and on and on. This type of negative thinking will not only sabotage your weight loss efforts but will actually cause you to gain weight too.

Approaching weight loss from a place of love will allow you—maybe for the first time in your life—to emerge from the great big burden of guilt and shame you feel about your weight. Once you are free from these feelings, you can focus freely and completely on giving yourself the gift of health.

How the Love Diet Came to Be

As a registered dietitian with a doctorate degree in nutrition and twenty years' experience at the Culinary Institute of America, my goal has always been to open readers' eyes to the bounty of incredible, healthful foods that can be used to create flavor and promote weight loss. In *The Sonoma Diet* (my *New York Times* bestseller, first published in 2005 and updated in 2010), I presented a successful weight loss protocol that introduced a new level of consciousness about food and flavor. But it wasn't until I started working on this book that I came face-to-face with the other critical factors that contribute to the overweight epidemic, factors that rest more on the medical and psychological side of the issue rather on the diet side. And this is where Dr. Dedomenico and his groundbreaking work with 20/20 LifeStyles come in—his comprehensive approach to weight loss addresses all these factors, and it's proven to produce unparalleled success.

I've worked with Dr. Dedomenico and his team of physicians, registered dietitians, certified exercise professionals, and psychologists for twenty years. Over this time, the 20/20 LifeStyles clinic has produced thousands of weight loss success stories. Many of these people were just like you—they had struggled with diet confusion and an imperfect dieting system for years, some for decades. At the clinic, they were finally able to change course. They were given the tools and guidance to change their lifestyles, behaviors, and habits. These patients not only lost weight, but they also learned to respect and love themselves, a process that has proven critical to losing weight and keeping it off. Research at 20/20 LifeStyles revealed that individuals who developed self-respect and self-love experienced lower stress hormone levels, diminished levels of whole-body inflammation, and significant weight loss; these individuals experienced both psychological and physiological benefits.

The numerous personal stories gave us insights into successful weight loss. We weren't just guessing what works or testing theories in a lab—we were seeing success happen in real people, in real life, right in front of us. We witnessed people like Donna who had been struggling with dieting for decades and lost sixty-four pounds, or Rage who overcame a binge-eating disorder to finally drop 108 pounds, and Renee who worked through issues with emotional eating to lose twenty-five pounds. Their weight loss only tells part of the story. Perhaps even more important is that they, along with many others who've attended the clinic, have been able to maintain their weight loss. The rate of success was astounding, especially when compared to the dismal numbers typically associated with other diets. Something was clearly going right.

Dr. Dedomenico and I realized that the overwhelmingly successful methodologies employed at 20/20 LifeStyles shouldn't just be available to those fortunate enough to live close to the clinic in Bellevue, Washington. Hence *The Love Diet* was born.

How *The Love Diet* Can Help You

This book is not like other diet books. That is because we focus on the whole *you*. It is not just about the food, calories, and exercise; it is also about your emotional attitude and well-being. If there's a tiny voice inside your head right now saying, "But I'm not worth it," or "This won't work for me," read on, because this book will change your life.

You will learn how to let go of blame. Blame is self-defeating. It leads to feelings of guilt and shame. This causes you to give up on yourself and, in many cases, not like yourself. Placing blame, whether it's on yourself or others, is an exercise in defeat. Instead of producing solutions or solving anything, blame just leaves you stuck in one place. People who have repeatedly struggled with weight most often blame themselves. It's not uncommon for that blame to join forces with feelings of shame and guilt and for all the negativity to ball up into one giant heap of resignation: *I don't like myself.* But that thought can change—and it must—for you to succeed. It all starts with letting go of guilt, blame, and shame. We'll teach you how it's done.

You will gain a restored confidence in the dietary choices you make—and in yourself. The Love Diet is based upon proven nutritional strategies that have been used for years at the 20/20 LifeStyles clinic. You won't be a diet guinea pig but instead will benefit from the rigorously researched and clinically solid practices that routinely produce lasting weight loss in people just like you. When you follow the guidance offered to you in this book, you will lose weight and keep it off.

The diet portion of the book will introduce you to the Seven Stages, an elimination diet designed to set you up for optimal success. You will first be given a dietary foundation and then we will help you to build upon it as you reintroduce foods to your daily meals, ultimately leading you to a way of eating that you can stick with for the rest of your life.

The Seven Stages begin with higher protein intake and a controlled quantity of healthy fats and carbohydrates. Gradually, specific food groups will be added back into your meals, allowing you to identify any reactions you might have to certain foods, such as digestive discomfort, inflammation (e.g., joint pain), and even skin rashes.

You will discover sustainable practices that come together to create a lifestyle, not a passing phase. The Love Diet is not a fad diet. The program you will encounter here takes a 360-degree view of what it means to lose weight in real life. It's not just about a clinically solid, comprehensive eating plan (though you will get this too), but it's also a new awareness of the other influences in your life. Your daily habits, your relationships with family members and significant others, how you talk to yourself, how you were raised, and how you were taught to eat—all of these factors influence who you are and how successful you are with sticking to a healthy lifestyle. We'll help you address the backstory so that you can create a new story.

You will see what success looks like in real people. If you've struggled with your weight for a long time or have a significant amount of weight to lose, it's easy to feel alone and isolated by this struggle. People who are of a healthy weight don't always understand what it's like, and even those who diet to lose ten pounds for special occasions don't *really* get it. But there are people who do. And a lot of them have passed through the doors at 20/20 LifeStyles and emerged on the other side with incredible and inspiring stories to tell. In *The Love Diet,* you will get to meet them and read about the very real problems that stood in their way and how those problems were solved. And more importantly, you will learn how these solutions will help you with your own weight loss issues.

Love Is All You Need? Not Quite

Of course, there is no Love Diet without the *love*—and restoring or establishing positive and compassionate feelings toward yourself will be central to your success in this program. If you're leery of the love talk, that's okay—at first, many of the individuals who would go on to become standout success stories were too. It's not common to see the terms *weight loss* and *love* discussed together, which is a great disservice to the millions of people struggling to achieve a healthy weight. But self-love is often the missing part of the equation for success.

Yet, the Love Diet isn't just about self-love, nor is it an overly sentimental guide to nutritional healing. Instead it is a proven guide to permanent weight loss written *by* people who know why diets fail and *for* people who are tired of the endless dieting cycle and want to lose weight for good. If you've never dieted before, you're also in luck—this can be your first and final avenue to dieting success.

We've written this book to give you the opportunity to become the *you* you've always wanted to be. Now is the time to make it happen.

PART I

Meet the Love Diet: A Brand-New Perspective on Losing Weight

CHAPTER 1

What's Love Got to Do with It?

You've picked up this book because you want to lose weight. And you've wanted—and struggled—to lose it for years. What started as a few extra annoying pounds has, year after year, turned into a lot of extra pounds. Physically, the weight is taking its toll. Maybe your joints have begun to ache more or your cholesterol levels and blood pressure continue to rise. Or maybe your doctor has diagnosed you with prediabetes or—worse—type 2 diabetes, the chronic condition that impairs your body's ability to use insulin to balance blood sugar levels.

Your weight affects you emotionally and socially too. At its worst, your weight might also be interfering with how you live your life: maybe you've skipped parties because you're worried you won't feel comfortable in any of your clothes, or maybe you've stressed about the need to squeeze into a booth at a restaurant, or maybe you've worried that your body might spill out of the narrow confines of an airplane seat. You spend time wishing you could run around with your kids or walk miles at an amusement park with ease. You constantly wonder if anyone will find you attractive again, even though you wouldn't dare to pay yourself a compliment.

When you stop to add up all the time you spend thinking about your weight for whatever reason—whether it's stressing over numbers on the scale or searching for and trying the latest diet trend—you realize—whether you wanted it to or not—your weight has become the main focus of your life.

My weight has become the main focus of my life.

When you say it out loud, do you find yourself nodding in agreement? If you do, you are not alone. In fact, nearly 200 million people in this country are right there with you. Two out of three people in the United States are saddled with weight issues. We have become an overweight nation with overweight habits and an overweight mentality that has consumed our way of life.

The health consequences are serious. New research shows that the root cause of type 2 diabetes is found in fat cells, so we know that excess weight sets you up to develop the disease. Statistics show that there are almost 106 million people with type 2 diabetes and prediabetes in the United States, and each year 2 million more Americans are diagnosed with the disease. Excess weight, especially in the abdominal region, is also linked to metabolic syndrome, which significantly increases risk for heart disease, stroke, certain types of cancer, and more.

Yet, as damaging as weight gain is to the human body, its psychological cost is perhaps equally as damaging, as is its accompanying negative self-image. People with weight issues frequently have a severely negative self-perception, a low self-esteem that is driven by feelings of shame, guilt, and self-criticism. Those negative feelings and thoughts don't just evaporate into thin air—they become part of who you are, seeping into your everyday existence and establishing the foundation from which you act, eat, think, and feel. A negative self-worth is powerful enough to initiate a tendency to overeat and to introduce other habits that perpetuate weight gain. It's powerful enough to override even the best of intentions to make healthy, good-for-you choices.

What's incredible, though, is that the reverse is equally as powerful, if not more so. People with positive self-esteem make choices reflective of this positivity—they are kind, compassionate, thoughtful, and respectful of themselves. They treat their *self* the way they would treat someone else they care deeply about. When you develop a positive sense of self, your actions follow suit—it doesn't feel like a struggle to make positive choices for your health, body, and life; it feels like the natural and right thing to do for someone you love. That's why learning to love yourself is the most important process you will discover in this book. When you build a foundation of love, all the other parts will fall into place. But don't take our word for it—let's look at Donna's story to see how a question of love changed her life.

A Spark of Hope

Like so many others, Donna was desperate to end her long battle with dieting, but she had no idea where to turn. She had been dieting since she was a teenager, self-conscious at five feet one and 145 pounds. She was acutely aware of the fact that she didn't look like other girls in class, the girls who caught the attention of boys, the girls who could fit in the tiny athletic shorts required for PE.

Noticing that she was unhappy and struggling with self-confidence, her parents offered to help, standing by Donna as she tried every national weight loss program available. But Donna never made it through the first week. Every time she failed, her hope dwindled as her self-loathing grew. She was stuck on a frustrating weight loss journey, which seemed destined to never end.

By the time she was in her midthirties, Donna was five foot three and 180 pounds with a soft, prematurely aged appearance: even though she was in her early thirties, most people pegged her ten or fifteen years older. She hadn't gone to a gym in years and was seriously out of shape. Worst of all, Donna had resigned herself to never changing and considered herself permanently single, lonely, and unhappy.

Her doctor told her that her blood pressure had gone up to the point where she had to either go on medication or lose weight and she needed to lose fifty to sixty pounds. Donna wasn't surprised, but she felt hopeless—how could she lose weight this time when all the other times she had failed?

Compounding her troubles, Donna had also recently gone on a blind date that left her feeling down. Hours spent shopping for a dress that made her feel good were wasted on a guy who left the date early to "care for his sick mother." Between being ditched midmeal and dwelling on her weight—and now medical—issues, Donna couldn't muster much hope for a better future. Her morale was at an all-time low.

But one evening something happened that would change the course of her life. Her physician gave her a note to see Dr. Dedomenico at the 20/20 LifeStyles clinic. At the time, she thought nothing of it. She'd been on every diet known to humankind with little lasting success—why would she call this place and expect anything other than failure?

Yet, when she happened upon the doctor's note on a later Friday evening, she was struck by a small spark of hope. Could the note be a doorway to the future?

She called the number on the sheet of paper, and to her surprise a gentleman answered. It was Dr. Dedomenico. He was friendly and welcoming, and he wondered why she hadn't called sooner. Donna seized the moment to be completely honest.

"Doctor," she said, "I didn't call because I didn't want to live through another failure. I just couldn't stand that. I've been overweight since I was five. I've been on every diet I could find, but it hasn't done any good. I'm a hopeless case."

"Donna, can I ask you something?"

She waited for the same old questions about her weight, what she ate, how often she exercised, and so on.

"Do you love yourself?"

Donna was shocked. She didn't know how to answer.

Dr. Dedomenico repeated the question. "I'm sorry. I hope you don't mind me asking. But . . . do you love yourself?"

Donna felt wary of a stranger asking such a personal question, but she couldn't help but contemplate the thought—she couldn't recall the last time she'd even considered the idea of loving herself.

"Honestly, it's been a very long time since I loved myself. I don't know where or when it went away, but it's gone. For years, I think I've been substituting food for love, and it hasn't worked. I don't even like myself."

Dr. Dedomenico wasn't stunned like she thought he might be. He said, "Donna, you're not alone. Many people we work with have felt exactly the way you do. And we've helped guide them toward liking—even loving—themselves again and toward a life filled with more happiness and health than they ever thought possible."

His words were so heartfelt that Donna's misgivings began to fade.

Donna's new story begins with that phone call. She entered the 20/20 LifeStyles program, and a new world opened to her. She learned that she really wasn't alone in her struggles—that there were people just like her all around. She learned how the stress and depression that she'd felt about her weight had actually caused her to gain more weight and that the food conditioning she'd been subject to growing up had established in her an unhealthy relationship with food. She learned about the harm she'd been causing her body. Although she'd known she'd been destroying herself for quite some time, she suddenly began to care about it.

Donna experienced nothing short of a complete transformation. She went from being depressed and hopeless to truly feeling like a brand-new person. The individual who felt like a failure, swimming in feelings of shame, guilt, and self-loathing, vanished. In her place emerged an optimistic, determined, and confident woman.

Now, nearly five years later, this new version of Donna is still around, living a rich life filled with health and love, and happier than ever. She became a runner and recently completed her first half marathon. She exercises three days a week, her blood pressure is normal, and she weighs 116 pounds, a lot of which is muscle. Her closet is free of oversized, tent-shaped shirts and is now full of form-fitting dresses that make her look and feel great. Donna has a new problem, though: when she goes shopping, everything fits and looks great and, as a result, she's become a clotheshorse. But that's okay—she has plenty to wear on date nights with her new husband.

The Path to Love

When you read through Donna's story, did you recognize any similarities to your own life? You don't have to have experienced a disappointing blind date to know what rejection or low self-esteem feel like. You don't have to have been dieting since you were a teenager to understand the frustration associated with weight loss failure or to have lost confidence in any program that promises success. Importantly, you don't have to identify with Donna to re-create her success in your own life.

But chances are you do identify with her, whether you know it or not. Chances are, just like Donna and the thousands of others with whom we've worked, something is missing from your life, even if you

THE LOVE DIET + 20/20 LIFESTYLES CONNECTION

The principles in *The Love Diet* are based on the very same ones used at 20/20 LifeStyles, a highly successful weight loss clinic located in Bellevue, Washington. Started by Dr. Dedomenico in 1992, the clinic has helped thousands of people overcome the imperfect dieting system and put them on the path to permanent weight loss. The medically based program used there helps restore metabolic balance, which is crucial to producing weight loss and to helping reverse risk for diseases such as type 2 diabetes and heart disease.

The clinic offers one of the most successful weight loss programs in the country—yet for many years, our insight on dieting success was only available to those willing to travel to the Bellevue location. When we considered the rise in weight-related diseases and the overwhelming number of individuals struggling with weight problems, we knew it was time to distill our program principles into a book format and make it available to all. The result is the book you're reading right now. It's your turn to experience success!

can't pinpoint what it is. Something so profound that its absence can undermine any and all efforts you make to create positive changes in your health habits and your life (because without it, you will always feel undeserving of the rewards). That something is love, of course. It wasn't until Donna developed love for herself that she was able to build the rest of her dream life around it. The Love Diet will put you on the same path.

You might find it difficult at this point to understand how love relates to weight loss—and that's okay. Our goal in this book is not only to help you understand how love influences and informs your motivation to take care of yourself but to also help you discover the many aspects of your life that contribute to how successful you are with a weight loss program (or any goal pursuit). Learning to love yourself is a process, and it requires stepping back to look at these other aspects in play—guilt, shame, blame, food conditioning, genetics, family dynamics, and more can impact your ability to lose weight. You may not even be aware of how powerful some of these forces are in your life, but they are there and can be more destructive than you realize. Shining a light on patterns of guilt, shame, and the other underlying influencers will help us illuminate the path to love. Let's explore further.

Food Is Not Love: Breaking the Shame Cycle

Have you ever overeaten and felt guilty and ashamed, then found yourself wanting to eat more to deal with these feelings? But instead of feeling better after eating, you only felt a deeper sense of guilt and shame, and even began to feel depressed? If so, you've fallen into the Shame Cycle, a whirlwind of overeating and emotions that over time can drag you into self-defeat, long-term depression, and extreme hopelessness. The cycle is fueled internally by biochemical changes that occur when you begin to feel depressed, namely by the increase of cortisol, which makes you hungry and can promote weight gain. Here's what the Shame Cycle looks like:

Overeating → Guilt and Shame → Emotional eating → Depression ← Depression increases cortisol ← Cortisol makes you hungry ← Weight gain → Hopelessness →
SHAME CYCLE

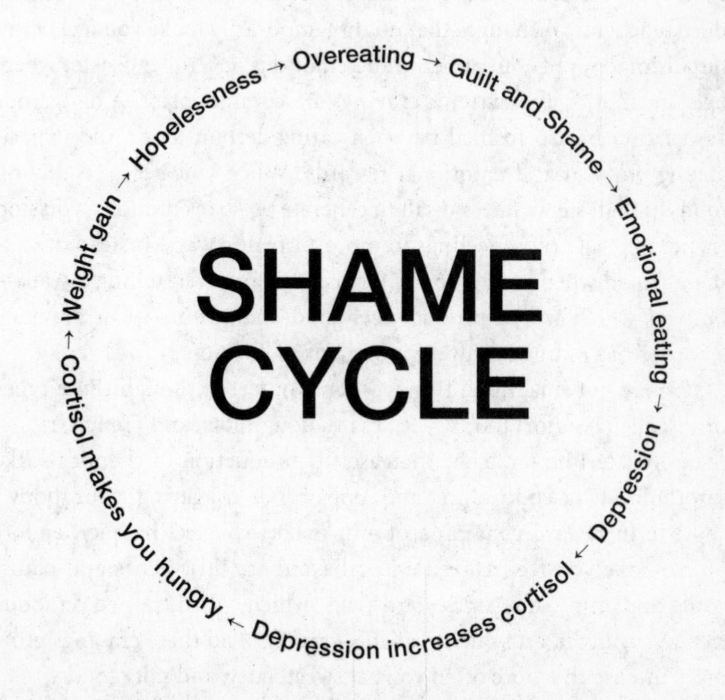

Guilt and shame aren't the only triggers of emotional eating. In fact, many people are driven to eat because they feel unwanted, unimportant, or unloved. They don't turn to food as a coping mechanism because it's sensible or logical but usually because it's what they've been taught to do. If you find yourself reaching for food to deal with feelings, you might have learned at a very young age that food is love or that it can be used for comfort, celebration, and companionship. Twenty, thirty, or forty years later, the relationship between food and feelings remains, despite the fact that food will never satiate a hunger for love or other fulfilling emotions.

A large percentage of people with weight problems have internalized the food-is-love message, unknowingly establishing a pattern of behavior and an emotional environment that begets and reinforces low self-esteem. When you use food as love, this process becomes a substitute for learning to love yourself directly.

The types of foods we gravitate toward when we're feeling bad only exacerbate the problem. Foods that are high in fat, sugar, and salt produce biochemical changes that might temporarily make you feel better but ultimately put your appetite and emotions on a roller coaster where extreme moods and extreme cravings are commonplace. A dangerous association is also formed between eating certain foods and experiencing physical and emotional rewards. When you begin to rely on foods high in sugar, fat, and salt to generate positive emotions, you stop trying to create those feelings in more authentic ways. Instead of calling a friend when you're down, for instance, or even taking a walk—both of which would produce feel-good endorphins—you gravitate toward a bag of unhealthy chips or a box of cookies.

You're not imagining things when you feel as though these types of so-called comfort foods—i.e., pizza, doughnuts, and French fries—make you feel better. They increase the production of chemicals like serotonin, beta-endorphin, and dopamine, triggering your body's short-term reward center. Serotonin makes you feel happier, endorphins make you feel relaxed and relieve those little aches and pains, while dopamine intensifies your focus, which, when trained on foods rich in sugar, fat, and salt, is called a craving. And these cravings grow more intense the more often you eat sweet, fatty, and salty foods.

The problem is these feel-good bursts don't last and they most certainly don't come for free. They encourage you to eat when you're not hungry or to eat too much and, eventually, to chronically consume too many calories each day. The result is steady and sometimes sneaky weight gain—before you know it, you're fifty pounds overweight.

The Blame Stops Here

It's easy to feel as though you should blame yourself for overeating and the consequence of excess weight. And yet there are so many factors stacked against you. First off, food manufacturers, fast-food companies, and restaurant chains are aware of the addictive quality of sugar, fat, and salt, and they aren't afraid to capitalize on it. They engineer foods specifically to get you hooked and keep you coming back for more—the more you consume, the more money they make. Even foods that are labeled as *diet, light, low fat, sugar-free,* and *gluten-free* are usually loaded with unhealthy calories.

Adding to the problem is the lack of reliable, trusted resources on matters involving nutrition and weight gain. Most doctors do not have the time to advise their patients on the proper protocols to lose weight and keep it off for good.

The good news is you'll find the guidance you need in this book. As you continue to read *The Love Diet,* you will discover not only nonjudgmental, compassionate direction but also a complete and proven nutritional plan that will help you as much as it's helped the thousands of people before you.

For each of those individuals, an important starting point on the path to success was letting go of self-blame and the shame and guilt that came along with it. Like you, they had to be alerted to all of the factors influencing their struggle with weight loss and the frustrating trappings of the shame cycle. Only by discovering the ways that the cards are stacked against you and becoming aware of the shame cycle can you then begin to break free from the patterns that have kept you stuck for so long.

The most important first step is to acknowledge that self-blame is self-destructive. Only then can you work toward removing it altogether. When you remove self-blame, guilt, and shame from your life, you make room for self-acceptance and self-love to enter and start to build the foundation of permanent weight loss. This process is part of something that we call adopting a Slimming Mindset, a central part of the Love Diet.

The Slimming Mindset

In our work at 20/20 LifeStyles, we have confirmed that guilt and shame can only be resolved through self-acceptance, which leads to self-respect and self-love. Loving yourself is the ultimate goal. When you love yourself, it feels natural and easy to make choices that are good for you and best for your body; you begin to treat yourself with the respect you deserve. When you have successfully begun to care enough about yourself to take care of your *self,* you have successfully adopted a Slimming Mindset. Adopting the mindset requires that you take the following steps:

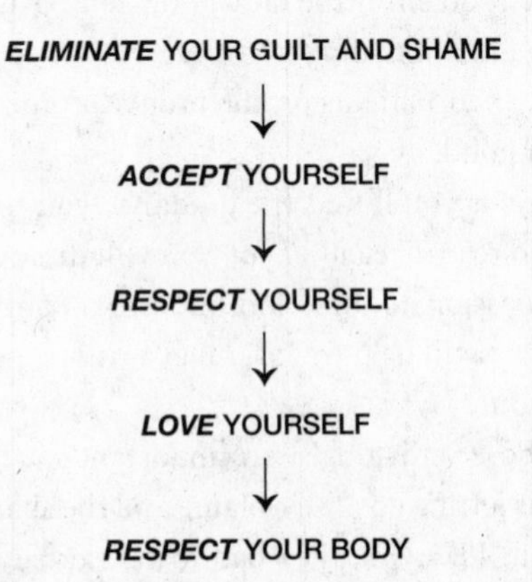

We have seen that self-respect and self-love can only occur after self-acceptance. Self-love cannot exist in someone who feels guilt or shame. The first step, then, in achieving self-love is to resolve the guilt and the shame.

You've learned that a critical part of letting go of guilt and shame is eliminating blame. It's time to officially free yourself from the critical, harsh judgments you place on yourself for overeating, gaining weight, or staying overweight—they're not productive or helpful to you, and they will continue to prevent you from achieving your goals. Even the little amount of knowledge you've gained thus far in *The Love Diet* will help release the chains of self-blame. You've already discovered that it's not your fault. You've already learned that you deserve a clean slate.

To work toward self-love, you must begin to *act as if.* That means you have to act like people who respect and love themselves. People who love themselves have treating themselves well down to a science; they don't have to force healthy habits related to eating and exercise. They practice these habits because they see themselves as worthy of the rewards. Try this approach on for size, letting your actions come from a place of caring and love. If you do this long enough, your behavior starts to become automatic.

Operating from love also means making room for forgiveness. If you gained five pounds and none of your clothes fit, or you started your diet at 7:00 A.M. and you've blown it by 5:00 P.M., do you resume beating yourself up? No. Loving yourself includes giving yourself permission to make mistakes. This is called applying the doctrine of unconditional acceptance. Acceptance of who you are is not contingent upon perfection. The truth is that nobody is perfect.

It's time to face the fact that you are an imperfect being. We all are. It now becomes your goal to accept yourself unconditionally and strive for improvement. As with any skill, the more you practice self-acceptance, the better you will become at it, and the stronger your love for yourself will grow.

Once you feel self-love, the world automatically becomes a better place. In fact, you feel so good that you delight in being kind and generous to yourself. You will no longer feel nondeserving. You will strive for goals without fear of failure. You will begin to treat your body in a loving way, which leads to better health. You will successfully lose weight, maintain your weight loss, and improve your physical condition, which will lead to a healthier, happier, and longer life.

There's an added benefit too: once you learn to love yourself, you'll be amazed at how much love you receive from others.

An Exciting Opportunity

You might have noticed by now that *The Love Diet* takes an unconventional approach to weight loss. Rather than simply jumping right into a discussion on calories or what you'll be eating, we have focused first on establishing an awareness of some of the psychological factors that have helped produce your issues with weight. Our clinical work with thousands of people has shown that this is the only reliable path to permanent weight loss. Of course what you eat and how much is an essential part of the plan as well, and the next chapter will give you a preview of what's to come in the Seven Stages, our rigorously researched and tested diet portion of the book.

Before you move on to the next chapter, however, we'd like to make sure you're fully ready and open to what *The Love Diet* has to offer. An essential part of being ready is making sure your mind is in the right place. Like many of the people we've helped at 20/20 LifeStyles, you may be in a place of doubt—you may find yourself reading through these pages with every intention of trying the plan, but there's still this voice in the back of your head saying, "This isn't going to work. Nothing else has—why would this be any different?" If you're going to be successful, you have to change your mindset; you have to approach the program with an open mind.

A closed mind is your own personal prison. When you feel hopeless, it's easy to convince yourself that there's no solution—this self-defeating form of reassurance is what's known as a closed loop. When you're in a closed loop, you eliminate any chances to take in new information or reanalyze your situation—and this is when you truly do become stuck. This process is terribly self-defeating, but it also happens to be somewhat comfortable. Why? Because there's no risk. There's no anxiety about trying out new experiences. There's no apprehension about learning new things. There's no fear of failure. You've locked yourself up in a strangely comfortable prison, but it's a prison nonetheless. The only way out is to confront the anxiety of trying and learning new things. That breakthrough can be uncomfortable. Yet granting yourself the gift of openness and the power to persevere can open the doors to a truly transformative experience.

So how do you prevent fear from keeping you in prison? Well, in this case, fear is related to two perceptions:

1. What others think of you
2. What you think of yourself based on what they think of you

When you lock yourself into this opinion-driven fear, you are essentially trapping yourself in a box built from fleeting illusions. The opinions of others, even if they match up with what you imagine them to be—which is rarely the case—are temporary. Other people's opinions have only as much power as you give to them: if you empower them, they will imprison you.

But freedom is always one choice away. When you make the choice to accept yourself, which you do when you absolve yourself of any guilt and shame you have around your eating habits and weight, you become more powerful than any opinions, any judgments. You don't just unlock the door to the prison—you break it down. And you officially open up your life to a new destiny.

As you prepare to dig into the dietary details of *The Love Diet*, it's important to be truly open to a new and different outcome for yourself on the other side of this plan. It's time to stop telling yourself and accepting the same "I'm a diet failure." In your hands, you hold the path to a new story with a different ending. If you close your eyes, you can see the future you: you're happy, healthy, full of energy, unburdened by excess weight, and making the choices each day that will give you the life you deserve.

Now, let's make that future a reality!

CHAPTER 2

Ready, Set, Go! Creating and Supporting Your Trigger Moment

Think of someone in your life who has made a change. Maybe you have a parent who quit smoking, a friend who made a career change, or perhaps it was you who turned over a new leaf and became a saver instead of a spender.

In all of these cases, the path to making a change wasn't a simple one; it involved many stops and starts. Even habits that come to an end by the so-called cold turkey method have a long mental history behind them, with months or even years of internal debates likely to have been waged.

This is the truth about change that no one tells you: it doesn't have an on-off switch. Instead, as researchers of human behavior have revealed, change is a process that involves a series of steps. Just like a caterpillar transforms into a butterfly through a series of stages, so do humans take a set path to improvement. We go through what's referred to as the Stages of Change, which take us from precontemplation, contemplation, preparation, action, and eventually maintenance.

It can look something like this: In the beginning, murmurs of consideration begin to bubble up, but are usually pushed down—"My doctor said I should lose weight, but I have a lot on my mind right now. I'll think about that later" (precontemplation). Then the tone shifts a bit: "Maybe I do want to lose weight; I wonder what my life would look like if I were healthier?" (contemplation). From there it's all about finding a plan and preparing to start: "*How* am I going to make this change happen?" (preparation). Next the plan is implemented and followed (action), naturally with some slipups here and there, and suddenly (or not quite so suddenly), new habits are in place (maintenance).

Most diet books and programs drop you right into the middle of action without ensuring that you're emotionally ready or adequately prepared to follow through with lifestyle changes. Unfortunately, this is all too often a setup for failure. At 20/20 LifeStyles, we see people every day who've tried many of these other diets and failed. Few of them stop to consider that the programs they've been following might have been what was inadequate rather than their own abilities.

Like those who've come to our clinic and experienced success, as a reader of *The Love Diet,* you will benefit from our 360-degree approach to permanent weight loss. This includes the vital exercise of reestablishing love for yourself, but another essential part of the process is acknowledging that it is in fact a process made up of several steps—learning about these steps and about how change works will give you an advantage in making the process happen in your own life.

As you read through this chapter, think of yourself as having just discovered a secret treasure map with directions to permanent weight loss success. Your awareness of each stage of change will put you that much closer to achieving your goal. We'll be your guides along the way, helping you develop an understanding of the stages and providing specific action items—see the sections called Push Yourself Forward—that will put you in control of your progress.

Getting to Know the Stages of Change

You can overhaul your eating and exercise habits by getting acquainted with the stages, identifying where you might be in the process, and then using this awareness to help steady you for the next step. Don't get discouraged if you find that you're at the very beginning—every stage is valuable and necessary, and regardless of where you find yourself, you are making progress toward change. The goal now is just to keep going.

Here's a more detailed look at the stages and how you can push forward no matter where you are in the process:

Precontemplation is when you avoid the problem or pretend it doesn't exist; it's likely where you were before you decided to read this book (which means you deserve a congratulations for getting to this point all on your own!). In precontemplation, you eat whatever you want whenever you want and however much you want. You aren't concerned about the consequences of these actions, and yet in the background you're spending considerable energy avoiding thoughts about what you are doing to your body. You rationalize, deny, or simply avoid looking at the issue completely. Precontemplation comes with a healthy dose of denial. Suggestions from a spouse, friend, or doctor to work on your weight are not welcomed, and the conversations are likely to take a prickly turn. Simply put: you're not ready, but inside something is brewing.

Push yourself forward: Again, since you've already picked up this book, you're beyond the precontemplation stage. But just to be sure you continue to build momentum, we want you to start thinking about the benefits of losing weight and getting healthy. Focus on the positives of living a healthier lifestyle instead of what you perceive to be the difficulties of getting there. There's an endless supply of good things coming your way.

Contemplation is the next stage, and if you're here, you've lost the ability to avoid thinking about your weight problem. You have accepted that there is a problem, but you're not sure what to do about it. The good news is you're open to solutions and seeking stories of success. It's this openness that led you to pick up this book and to create change in your life. You're less concerned with the cons and focusing more on the pros and benefits you'll experience as a result of the changes you're about to make. It's an exciting time—you're on the verge of making big shifts in your life.

Push yourself forward: We encourage you to read the success stories throughout these pages. You're open and ready to see what success looks like. Can you envision yourself running a half marathon, like Donna did (page 11)? Or taking on a new hiking hobby like Kurt (page 176)? Reading about the circumstances or situations others overcame to create successful change can be inspiring and confidence building.

Next comes **preparation.** During preparation, you are seeking and decisively identifying your plan of action. Since you picked up *The Love Diet,* we know that you already have your plan in hand. Beyond that, the main focus is to ensure that your environment is ready to produce the results you want. This includes identifying and removing any obstacles to success—this could be physical obstacles, such as junk food in the house, or mental obstacles, which could include lingering self-doubt or even people in your life who might sabotage your efforts.

Push yourself forward: There are many steps you can take to help propel yourself into the next stage, Action. First off, you can pick a date on which you will start day one of the diet. This is an obvious way to give yourself a clear starting point. You can also take inventory and make sure you have everything you need to follow the program: a food scale, good shoes for exercise, a tool for tracking food, whether it's our 20/20 LifeStyles app or a journal, and so on. We'll recap everything you need starting on page 79.

Now is also the time you can start practicing some of what will soon be your new habits. You don't have to go all the way quite yet, but consider beginning to phase out soda while incorporating more water or swapping highly processed snacks for foods such as raw veggies or Greek yogurt. And maybe next time you dine at a restaurant, order a large, fresh salad with a lean protein such as chicken or fish instead of a pasta dish or a burger and fries. Keep in mind that there's no pressure to be perfect—this is just practice!

When you've reached the **action** stage, you are committed and on the path to losing weight and gaining health. Your personal wellness has become a priority, and you will be more excited than ever about the profound transformation you are about to experience. If you've entered the Action stage, congratulations! There's a lot of thinking and emotional work that comes before this, so arriving here is an accomplishment in and of itself. Take the time to acknowledge yourself for having the confidence to commit and then keep going—you've got a plan to follow!

It's important to remember the practice of unconditional acceptance. If you make bad decisions, don't feel alone in this—slipups or lapses into old habits aren't uncommon. Be kind to yourself, but also make sure to get right back on track.

Push yourself forward: Moving forward to maintenance means reaching a point where your healthy ways are part of your everyday lifestyle. To help with this, focus on building and strengthening the support systems around you. Look to bond with friends who lead healthy lifestyles, or find new ones who do. You can also look for social groups online—the Internet is filled with people who are committed to eating well and exercising, and most of them are willing and eager to share their secrets and strategies.

Once you've reached **maintenance,** you are practically an old pro at living a healthy lifestyle. You have practiced your new eating habits to the point that you don't have to think twice anymore about what's best for your body. You not only *know* what's best—you consistently choose to *do* what's best. You care for your health and wellness the way you care for the health and wellness of people you love—you have become a person worthy of your own compassion and love.

You may even find that during this stage, people start turning to you for guidance and commenting on your level of commitment. They might ask, "How did you lose the weight?" or say things like, "I wish I had your willpower," which is when you can explain that it's all part of the process, or rather the Stages of Change. Think of how incredible this moment will feel.

Push yourself forward: Maintenance is really just the final nail in the coffin of your old lifestyle. Throughout the maintenance stage (we'll give you a specific maintenance plan in Chapter 13), you will overcome obstacles and learn to stick to your new habits even during challenging times. And each time you do this, you will build your confidence until you reach a point where your unhealthy habits will be nothing more than a part of your history.

You Can Do It: Making Change Happen

Now that you've learned about the Stages of Change, can you identify where you are today? Can you see the path you're going to take as you follow the program in *The Love Diet*? No matter where you are in the progression, you can feel proud of the fact that you are on your way.

We've found that each person remembers the moment when they went from contemplation to preparation and then on to action. The moment they would define as a trigger moment, during which they experienced a jolt of confidence and confirmation—the moment they were able to say, "I'm doing this. I'm going to change my life." Has that moment already arrived for you? Or is it just around the corner?

Let's take a look at Diana's story to see how her trigger moment spurred her into making a change.

As Diana describes it, the evening of change arrived with a sudden shift in her perception. She experienced what she could only describe as an "aha moment," which allowed her to see her life from an entirely different perspective.

She remembers it clearly. She was in the living room after dinner. Her three kids were off in their rooms getting ready for bed. She was in an armchair sipping a beer, and she glanced across the room at her husband, Don, who was sprawled out on the couch, also with a beer in hand. Suddenly, it hit her like a slap in the face: she was living her life entirely according to what he wanted. Everything they did was driven by Don's desires, not hers.

Her husband expected her to drink, and so drink she did. In fact, they couldn't have a conversation without alcoholic beverages in hand. As she gazed over at him on the couch, where he always was, she saw him with fresh eyes: he was drunk, his belly was hanging out, and he was grazing on potato chips as he watched sports on TV.

In that instant, her life began to come into focus. She thought about how since she had been a young girl, she had been a people pleaser, especially when it came to men. And she had another depressing thought: she and Don had sat together like this every evening for as long as she could remember, and this was likely how her evenings would be spent for years to come.

Diana felt frightened by this thought. There had to be more to life than this. She was struck by the idea of escape, suffocated by the thought of having to stay where she was. She actually jumped to her feet once and then abruptly sat down again, not knowing what to do. Glued to the TV, Don was oblivious to her unease, and as the minutes passed, she finally worked up the courage to speak.

"I think I need a change," she said.

"Huh?" He continued to stare at the screen.

"I said, I need a change in my life."

"That's nice, honey."

She raised her voice. "You're not listening to me."

Having gotten his attention, she told him that she wanted to do something new for herself. She was too fat, she said, and she knew it. What she couldn't say then was that she was also tired of trying to keep up with his alcoholic habits. Drinking had dominated their lives and caused frequent duress for herself and her kids.

She told Don that she wanted a different lifestyle and that she'd heard about a program that could help. He dismissed her with a wave of the hand and said she was probably just tired and would feel better in the morning. When she insisted that she was going to go sign up, he seemed threatened. What was he supposed to do with himself when she was away from home learning about the program?

Don peppered her with more questions, mostly about money. She said she had her own savings. Still, he complained further, getting angry about her wanting to do anything outside the home. There were too many responsibilities, he said. Why was she trying to make his life more difficult? he asked. She listened to his arguments and rants, but when she insisted on joining the program, he got suspicious. He suggested that she might be having an affair.

Diana denied the accusation as ridiculous because it was—she simply wanted to do something for herself. She wanted to focus on her own health for once and to look good again. She was nearly fifty pounds overweight and had a hard time feeling attractive. "I just want to be beautiful again," she said to Don. "I need to change."

"You're beautiful to me, and that's all that counts," he responded.

She knew she'd hit a brick wall. Her willingness to cater to her husband's wishes and years of spoiling him had put her in this spot. It finally hit her: her husband was an alcoholic, and to please him, she had become one too.

Don was right about one thing—there were too many jobs to do to run the household. She devoted no time or efforts to satisfying her own needs. She had a full-time job, three kids whom she cared for when she wasn't working, and a demanding man who had to have everything his way.

Her day usually began at 5:00 A.M., when she started to hustle to prepare breakfast for the family, get the kids off to school, get dressed, and arrive at work by 8:30. Then, after work, because it was part of the ritual, she would meet her husband at their favorite bar for several drinks at happy hour and maybe some dinner. Sometimes Don would hang out for more drinks or just follow her home, but either way, she would rush back to the house to feed her brood, ages nine, sixteen, and eighteen, by 6:00 P.M., and then do the rest of the kitchen cleanup and other housekeeping for the rest of the evening. The routine started all over again the next day.

Diana and Don continued to have a horrible argument that evening, all because she was ready to try to do something positive for herself. She was scared and confused, but after some soul-searching and contemplation, she finally called 20/20 LifeStyles and enrolled, knowing full well that her husband would be very upset.

When Diana started the program, the status quo of her marriage ended. After she began the Seven Stages, she tried to bridge the gap between her new habits and the old ones. She tried to stick with Don's alcoholic lifestyle despite the fact that she had started eating new meals and exercising. Any progress she made was neutralized by having to drink cocktails with her husband every evening to keep the peace.

In the meantime, Diana continued to work on herself. Counseling helped her to take an honest self-assessment and allowed her to begin to see why she was such a male-oriented woman. For one thing, Diana's mother had left home when she was four, and although Diana saw her on occasion, her mother really had no influence on her life. Her father had been a workaholic and, perhaps because his wife had deserted him, hypercritical of Diana as a female. Nothing Diana did was good enough, and she was made to feel inferior. Her dad was particularly disappointed at her lack of athletic ability and dissatisfied with anything but perfect grades. Diana tried her hardest to get all As because it was the only way to get a positive reaction from her dad.

Her willingness to please men expanded during puberty. She sought approval from her boyfriends, just as she had from her father. And the way she commanded attention was to find dysfunctional young men who depended on her for a number of things they couldn't or wouldn't do for themselves. Her mother, whom she still saw occasionally, called Diana the "bum magnet"—and it was true.

The day her "male bondage" ended was the day she defied her husband to sign up for 20/20 LifeStyles—this is the day Diana entered the action stage. After that, everything rotated 180 degrees. Where her identity had revolved around her husband's approval, the life lessons she learned while trying to lose weight convinced her that she was finally, for the first time, her own person in charge of her life. "I, alone," she would say to herself, "am responsible for the quality of my life." That statement defined her departure from male dependency.

The combination of dietary guidance, exercise, and counseling did wonders. Before, she would overeat the wrong foods because she allowed herself to get too hungry. Now, she was meal tracking, keeping her calorie counts in line, and exercising regularly.

She came to understand how distraught she'd been with the chaos created by the alcoholic culture of her marriage. As her mind began to open, she realized the utter lack of self-respect she'd had for herself—she had allowed others to discount her own feelings in decision making, and she'd been afraid to stand up for herself. When it came to food, she discovered that she had been a mindless eater, putting anything into her mouth without really tasting or enjoying. She now had the awareness that what she put in her mouth was fuel for her body and her mind. She was beginning to respect herself and her body.

Diana went on to lose nearly fifty pounds. She completely changed the shape of her body. She did eventually divorce her husband, and she became a new person—her old habits, feelings, and dependency were replaced with new feelings of hopefulness and independence. No longer was she pleasing everyone else at her expense; she was finally taking care of herself.

In Diana's story, we can see patterns of behavior that we see with a lot of people who come to our clinic. Many have out-of-balance priorities and a tendency to put themselves last, which can present a major roadblock on the road to change. When you're last on the list, feelings of self-worth and self-respect plummet, taking with them any motivation to change.

Can you see examples in your life where you're allowing yourself to be disrespected like Diana was? When you allow yourself to be disrespected or disregarded, you demonstrate a lack of love for yourself.

Fortunately, all it takes is a trigger moment to put you on the path to change. You can suddenly become aware of the reality of your life and your desperate desire for change; all it takes is opening your eyes to the truth. But seeing the reality and wanting to move forward aren't always enough—in some cases, there are obstacles that have to be eliminated before progress can be made. Diana, for instance, had to overcome her codependent relationship to her husband before she was truly free to improve her own life.

For others, the obstacles can be different—a sabotaging family member or friend or otherwise poor support system or an eating environment that prohibits healthy choices. Before you begin the Seven Stages, it's important to take inventory of your own life to see where potential roadblocks may lie. Having an awareness of these obstacles and developing a strategy to overcome them will be essential to your success once you begin the plan.

Getting the Support You Need at Home

Changing your lifestyle is challenging, and it can be even more so if you don't have a solid or positive support system. But you can remodel the system around you to make sure it doesn't leave you stuck in the contemplation stage or prevent your trigger moment from happening.

Some of you may have a wonderful built-in support system at home or might have people within your extended family to cheer you on as you work to create a healthier life for yourself. Others get this kind of encouragement from their friends. If you don't have family or friends around you, it might seem tough, but surprisingly this isn't the worst-case scenario. The toughest situation is when individuals are stuck in a tear-down system, in which the people around them make them feel

CODEPENDENCY: AN UNHAPPY STATE OF MIND

If you are codependent, you are so focused on pleasing others that you forget to consider taking care of yourself. If you're in a codependent relationship, you support someone else's dysfunctional behavior. This dysfunction can make you feel crazy, often bouncing you between feelings of submission and anger, most of which is directed at yourself. In a lot of cases, the anger feels seething and unsolvable; it's so constant that it pushes many toward food as a coping mechanism.

Codependents are normally created at a very early age. They're taught that everyone's feelings are more important than their own, that it's rude to ever say no. Codependents are criticized when their behavior isn't exactly the way their elders expect, even when those expectations aren't clear.

As a result, codependents feel they can do nothing right. They feel unworthy and believe they have no right to feel anything good or to express their own feelings. They try to fix everything in the family, their workplace, or their social group. When these attempts at social management fail, as they usually do, the codependent will feel angry and even more useless.

Obviously, being codependent doesn't give happiness a fair chance or make self-improvement a reality.

The answer isn't always to separate yourself completely from the person or people who trigger your codependent behavior. But rearrangements are in order. It's essential that the power structure of your family or social group be shifted to a more balanced state. Each individual needs to get at least some of their needs met, and they need to have some input into decisions that affect their lives. If you have always put yourself last and played a submissive, please-everyone role, you need to stand up and establish some new rules.

A conversation is a good place to start. Say: "I need to take care of myself too, which is why I'm making a commitment to improve my health. I hope you can support me just like I've always supported you." It's time to save some of your caring ways; stop giving them all away.

If Diana's story and this discussion on codependence resonated for you, we can recommend resources. Leaving codependent behaviors unaddressed can lead to frustrating experiences and dead-end attempts at personal change—in the end, you'll always come back to putting others first unless you work through your codependent tendencies. We encourage you to explore the Resource section for more information.

insignificant, unworthy, and unattractive. Are you surrounded by tear-down people? They are always in control, and they feel most secure when you are miserable.

When you think back to Diana's situation, you can see that she was living in a tear-down system. Her husband was controlling and demanding, discouraging Diana whenever she made an effort to focus on or better herself. He tore her down so that she wouldn't feel strong enough to stand on her own.

Hopefully, you aren't suffering in a similarly negative system. If you are, it's important to steel yourself before you reveal your plans for following the Love Diet. Be prepared to face criticism and questioning, as Diana did, but don't waver from your commitment. Remember that you are worth it, and know that the more focused and driven you become, the more drained and powerless the tear-down system will be.

Even in a supportive relationship, it's important to communicate and be open about your plans to change your habits. Since most couples and families share eating habits, if you're changing what you eat, your housemates might have to make some modifications on their end as well. Here are ways that you can set up your home environment and relationships for success:

- **Be an open book:** Others are more likely to be supportive when they understand what you're doing and how it will work. Share your concerns about your weight and the ways in which the Love Diet will help you finally regain control of your health.
- **Accentuate the positive:** Explain to your significant other and children why you're changing your habits and the benefits they'll get to experience as well—your weight will no longer hold you back or prohibit you from going places with them, nor will it continue to put your health at risk. This way you'll have cheerleaders, not complainers.
- **Invite everyone on board:** Set aside any feelings of guilt or shame you have about your weight and invite everyone to get on board your ship to success. This doesn't mean they have to follow the plan with you, but they can become active participants in your

progress. If you want your family to help with your nutrition, review the steps of the Seven Stages or share with them the core nutritional concepts you'll learn about in Chapter 4. This way, if someone else does the grocery shopping or cooking, they'll know what to pick up or make for you. Want an exercise or walking partner? Let your family know what days and what time you'll be heading out for your workout. You could even invite your significant other to follow the plan with you, if he or she is open to it.

Ultimately, as you work your way through the Stages of Change, communication is what matters most; don't be afraid to share the different feelings and thoughts that come up for you. And once you've begun the program, be clear about what's helpful and not helpful. Many of our participants with success stories shared examples of some supportive and not-so-supportive actions and behaviors implemented by their family members during the program. Take a look at these examples and share those that resonate with you about your family:

SUPPORTIVE ACTIONS:

- Removing junk foods from the house
- Keeping a positive attitude
- Being open to communicating about your process
- Acknowledging progress, whether it's weight loss or other improvements (e.g., better moods, less snoring, more energy)
- Offering to help with prepping healthful meals

NOT-SO-SUPPORTIVE ACTIONS:

- Hiding food
- Lecturing, criticizing, or reprimanding
- Being doubtful, judgmental, or impatient

It's important to keep in mind that this is most likely a new process for everyone involved. While it's imperative that your family understands what you're trying to accomplish, they also need to support you through each stage. When your family sees how committed you are to improving your health, they'll feel that much more supportive. Give them a reason to want to make some sacrifices in their own lives to help you.

If you get resistance on removing junk foods from the house, explain that it's healthier for the whole family to be eating more protein and veggies and fewer processed carbohydrates. Let them know how important it is to have nothing but healthful foods in the house—especially in the beginning when cravings or weak moments might make resisting junk foods even harder.

Early on, being home and eating at home will make it easier for you to stick to your plan. You can share with your family that during the first few weeks, you won't want to do too much traveling, dining out, or entertaining. Your commitment to the Seven Stages won't restrict your activities throughout, but this initial transformation will require discipline and a shift in your priorities. Think of yourself as an athlete, professional dancer, celebrity, or rock star preparing for that big opportunity—you are prepping yourself to look and feel amazing!

While certain activities and foods might get the boot (some just temporarily), new ones will take their place. Look for new activities and interests that aren't food focused but instead involve more physical activity. Think about going to play miniature golf with your kids or taking a hike with your significant other. Visit a museum or buy some new games to play. And ask your family to keep an open mind about trying new healthier foods and restaurants—if your health and weight are going to change, your eating and exercise habits have to change too. This is an undeniable fact.

"I, Alone, Am Responsible for the Quality of My Life"

While the people who surround you can inspire or discourage you as you approach and make changes in your life, they don't have the ultimate say in how you live your life: you do. It's essential for you to realize, like Diana did, that you are responsible for the quality of your life. Keep this in mind as you work to build support around you—and if you don't get the response you're hoping for initially, let this strengthen your love and commitment to yourself even more.

You can also seek support outside of your immediate home or family (this goes for people who are single too). Consider family members, friends, or coworkers as potential diet or support partners, especially those who might be also trying to overcome weight or metabolic issues. Or if you know someone who's successfully lost weight and kept it off, don't be shy about asking for their support and even mentorship—people who've achieved permanent weight loss are usually enthusiastic about sharing their knowledge and encouragement.

People who've never experienced weight challenges won't necessarily be unsupportive, but there are distinct aspects to your experience that they won't be able to fully understand. They've probably never experienced the type of metabolic imbalance that can torture you with crazy-making cravings and drive you to overeat. It's also unlikely that they can relate to the cycle of guilt and shame you feel about your weight and overeating, and your emotional state as you approach making this lifestyle change.

When you're searching for a compatible support partner or mentor, the most important thing is to be open and enthusiastic about engaging with others about your goal. You might find the best fit in someone close to you, maybe a sibling or another relative. Or perhaps a coworker, someone you know at church, or a book club or fantasy sports team member will want get on board with you. Either way, the best person will be someone who has dieted, or is dieting, successfully.

Having a support partner can help keep you accountable and make the process more fun and social. You'll find it's easier to exercise even on those days when you don't feel like it. And after you finish your plan, you can continue to encourage one another to exercise and expand your nutrition knowledge. Together, you can train toward completing an event, like a 5K race or a local hike or bike ride. We've found that many of our support partnerships do activities together: they share recipes, go shopping, take weekend hikes or bike rides, and dine out together. And these partnerships work well for both men and women, although we have found that in most cases, it works best when your support person is of the same sex. After you and your support partner have been together for a while, you might reach out and help another person.

The Choice to Make a Change

Modifying your health habits isn't easy, but it will be that much easier now that you know how change happens and what obstacles might get in your way. You have the knowledge that will help you identify where you are in the process and the tools to help push yourself forward—now it's just up to you to put the plan into action. If you've picked up this book after months or even years of lingering in the contemplative stage of change, let this moment be your trigger moment—there's no better time than right now to begin creating a better life for yourself.

CHAPTER 3

"Help—I Can't Stop!" How to Break Up with Overeating

Do you feel like you're always hungry? Have you ever eaten an entire box or bag of a food and not even noticed it until you were completely done? Do you wonder sometimes why you can't stop eating even when you want to?

If you answered yes to any of these questions, you are not alone. Overeating has become an all-too-common practice, and most people don't even realize the extent to which they do it. Nearly every individual who has entered our clinic has had to address the issue of overeating head-on. And whether it's involved emotional eating, mindless eating, or binge eating, we've helped guide them through it. In this chapter, we will show you how to break up with your own overeating habit.

Getting to the bottom of an overeating habit is an essential part of creating permanent weight loss. There are many contributing factors, and in some cases these factors can overlap one another and complicate the issue even further. For example, you could be prone to emotional eating—which will lead to the intake of excess calories—when you feel stressed, sad, or angry, but you could also eat a diet high in sugar, fat, and salt, all of which activate your reward center and compel you to eat far beyond fullness. When these overeating factors are in play and especially when they overlap, you are all but guaranteed to gain weight. That's because you don't have to eat much more than what your body needs for weight gain to happen—just 50 calories (half a slice of bread) beyond what you need a day can result in a weight gain of five pounds a year or fifty pounds in ten years.

SAYING GOODBYE TO FOOD HANGOVERS

Many of us eat the foods we love as a reward and then we feel terrible, which doesn't make much sense. And yet, we do it all the time. Why is it we overeat foods loaded with sugar, fat, and salt and then groan in physical discomfort, swearing never to do it again . . . only to repeat the same process days, even hours, later?

One explanation is that the immediate good feelings you get from foods containing sugar, fat, and salt are far more powerful in influencing your behavior than the misery you feel later. Foods such as chips, ice cream, pizza, and French fries provide immediate stimulation to the pleasure center in your brain. The punishment—when you wake up feeling tired and bloated and dealing with digestive distress—is delayed just enough that you no longer connect it to the food, the association between food and your physical discomfort having weakened over time.

The same behavior pattern happens with other addictive substances such as drugs and alcohol. That's because all these substances light up the reward center in our brains, triggering the release of serotonin, endorphins, and dopamine and creating a temporary pleasure high. It doesn't last, though, and despite the repercussions, you still want to go back for more. It's a vicious cycle! The only way to break the junk food addiction is to remove fast foods and other processed foods from your diet. While you might feel deprived initially, the long-term rewards will be so much greater than the temporary pleasure you've given up—you will experience freedom from cravings, increased weight loss, and more energy, and you never have to experience a food hangover ever again.

Resolving issues with overeating requires more than just trying out a new diet. You must dig a little deeper and get to the root of the problem before you can make new, healthier eating habits permanent. If you try to make more surface-level dietary changes without addressing these underlying factors, your struggles with weight are destined to continue.

Through research and work with thousands of individuals, we've identified three key factors that can set you up to overeat. They have to do with *what* you eat, *why* you eat, and *how* you eat. When it comes to what you eat, certain foods can disrupt hormones that influence appetite, preventing your body from receiving messages of fullness. Why you eat is all about emotions and eating intentions—are you eating to fuel your body or to soothe a feeling? This is a critical question to consider, and we'll help you answer it. How you eat has to do with your habits—are your habits programming you to be a mindless eater?

In this chapter, we'll delve a bit deeper into these underlying factors that can activate and perpetuate overeating. And more importantly, we'll include proven methods for addressing them so that they no longer sabotage your weight loss efforts. Let's take a look.

Is What You Eat Setting You Up to Overeat?

A steady diet of simple, refined carbs (you'll learn more about these in Chapter 4) can lead to chronically high insulin, which increases fat storage and accelerates weight gain. Once excess weight is on the body, other hormonal imbalances occur, which only worsen the situation by letting your appetite run wild.

One hormone vitally important to appetite control can be affected directly by weight gain. This hormone, leptin, is manufactured by the fat cells and travels to the brain to deliver a message of fullness. Leptin is your body's own appetite suppressant, and since it comes from fat cells, the more fat you have on your body, the more leptin will be produced. Similarly, the less fat, the less leptin (if you're too thin, your body will signal the need to eat more). In this way, your body works to help you maintain a set weight by ensuring that you don't over- or undereat. But it only works when your brain gets leptin's messages, and delivery failure can create big problems. Many overweight people develop leptin resistance, a state in which the brain stops responding to leptin and hunger is allowed to continue unchecked. Scientists believe this resistance develops when the body produces certain types of proteins that block leptin receptor sites in the brain. What triggers the production of these interfering proteins? Being overweight or obese, having high blood sugar, or having high insulin levels. You might be leptin resistant if you have any of these conditions or if you eat a high-fat diet. Lifestyle factors such as not getting enough sleep or having high levels of stress (see "The Love Diet Guide to Better Sleep and Less Stress" in the Resources section) can also lessen your leptin responsiveness.

To correct leptin resistance, we must look to what you eat. There are specific dietary strategies that, when applied, can actually make it easy for you to avoid overeating. Here are a few ways that you can take better advantage of your body's natural appetite suppressant:

- **Cut out sugary, simple carbs:** This will produce a trifecta of benefits by keeping blood sugar and insulin low and curbing fat storage (you'll read more about simple carbs and weight gain in Chapter 4).
- **Minimize high-fat foods:** These include processed snack foods and chips. Cutting them back will improve leptin sensitivity and help keep your appetite in check.
- **Avoid overly restrictive dieting:** You might be enticed by the rapid fat loss promised by very low–calorie diets, but be warned: it could backfire. If you lose fat too quickly, your body will begin to produce less leptin, leaving you fighting hunger and constant cravings.

When you begin following the Seven Stages, you will automatically start to apply these strategies to your diet. You'll also discover what foods you should be eating in place of those that can contribute to leptin resistance. Nutrient-rich vegetables and lean proteins, such as poultry, seafood, and leaner cuts of beef, will keep insulin and blood sugar low and help cut production of those leptin-interfering proteins. Healthy fats, such as extra-virgin olive oil, avocado, nuts, and canola oil, will provide a slow and steady source of energy without having a negative impact on your leptin sensitivity. Importantly, the plan will also provide enough calories to prevent leptin levels from plummeting too quickly, an event that could trigger extreme hunger and overeating.

The Million-Dollar Question: Why Are You Overeating?

When you think about your eating habits, it's important to consider why you eat. At the fundamental level, we all eat because food is what keeps us alive. But most of us don't just eat what we need to keep our bodies running and then stop. This is partly due to our overabundant food culture—we can't ever go too far without being reminded that we should be eating more. TV, radio, and magazine ads tell us what we should be putting in our mouths, and even roadside billboards suggest that we're missing out if we don't pull over immediately to try the latest and greatest fast-food creation. It's also due to the fact that people are increasingly engaging in emotional eating.

Most of the people who have come to our clinic are emotional eaters to some degree. They eat when they're angry, depressed, lonely, tired, or bored. Many even use food to generate or recall feelings of love, a connection they learned to make as children. While it's not unhealthy to connect eating with pleasure—nearly all of our holidays, family gatherings, and celebrations include food—it is a dangerous habit to use food in place of dealing with feelings. It is also a slippery slope. Once you begin to use food to cope with one type of emotion, it's not long before you use it to deal with other feelings. This is what happened with Angela, who came to us when she was fifty and ready to change her life.

When we first met with Angela, she explained that she felt like she'd lost contact with herself—she no longer knew who she wanted to be or how she should feel about her life. On the outside she seemed to function effectively, even leading a successful career as a prosecuting attorney, but on the inside she felt a complete mess. Years of career-related stress and the loss of her husband a few years earlier had left her in an uncertain state, and she was too anxious and overwhelmed to find a solution on her own.

With Angela, it was important to look to her past for clues on why she was feeling such severe emotional instability. Like many others, the roots of her confusion stemmed from childhood. She was raised by an alcoholic father and a narcissistic mother, and their dysfunctional dynamic had left her with a scarred self-esteem and a tendency toward self-destructive behaviors.

An alcoholic parent can create chaos in any household. In Angela's case, each day was a mystery: would she be seeing the fun dad today or the angry, raging monster? Angela's mother tried to compensate for her father's mental abuse by focusing on the future Angela would have, and she began grooming her to be perfect. Since the family was sick on the inside, Angela's mom wanted Angela to look perfect on the outside.

Unfortunately, her efforts to cover up the dysfunction turned extreme and she became hypercritical of Angela. She constantly criticized Angela's weight and even went so far as to have Angela take amphetamines to increase her weight loss. Looking back, Angela couldn't recall how many pills she had taken—they were too numerous to count.

It's also difficult to assess how much amphetamines distort the childhood learning process. For Angela, it seems to have affected her mental state dramatically, adding to the stress she already felt living in a constantly unpredictable environment.

Ironically, pictures of Angela as a little girl reveal that she was never fat. Her mother's efforts were clearly made in an attempt to take the focus off the real problem in the household: Dad's alcoholism. And Mom's misplaced efforts continued well into Angela's teens.

Angela had been taught at a young age that women must be very thin to have any worth. Countless women are taught this misconception growing up, and it's led to self-acceptance issues for most, if not all of them. The pressure to be thin can be overwhelming and lead to a willingness to try anything to lose weight, including dangerous fad diets that come with serious health risks.

Angela rebelled against her mother's tyranny the only way she knew how: by eating. She had been taught, after all, that food was an instrument of control. The more her mother tried to regulate her food, the more Angela ate. When Angela was frustrated, she would isolate herself to read books and eat. When she was lonely, she ate. When she was sad, she ate. When she was tired, she ate. Whenever she was enjoying herself, she ate. Food, not alcohol, became her drug of choice.

Her reliance on food and the habitual use of it for emotional support followed her into adulthood. And with the passage of time, Angela found herself significantly overweight. The excess weight created health problems, saddling her with chronic arthritis and insomnia as well as emotional problems, which only lowered her already shaky self-esteem.

Her lack of self-respect led to a long and destructive relationship with a man, and she felt lower than ever. She was stuck in a cycle of self-abuse, eating to comfort her emotional struggles and, later, smoking to deal with the constant stress she felt.

It seemed things were taking a turn for the better when Angela met and married a wonderful man. But that time was cut short when he died unexpectedly. His passing compelled Angela to relocate and try to start over with her life. A new town led to feelings of isolation and depression, which she once again tried to comfort with food.

Angela found her way to a new career as an ordained minister and developed a new group of friends, but she still felt unfulfilled and confused. Her weight gain and her depression contributed to a round of poor health, and she began to think more on the concept of the mind-body connection—would her body ever be at peace if her mind wasn't?

And this is when Angela visited our clinic. She was confused, lost, and unsettled emotionally but ready to create a change in her health and life. What she discovered at 20/20 LifeStyles (as you'll discover in this book) was a program that not only treated her sick body but, as she put it, healed her mind and soul as well. She learned that she was capable of delivering the love and respect she needed; it didn't have to come from food or through others.

As a Christian, Angela had always believed in a separation of the body and soul, with the soul being the focus and the body being simply a vessel. But what she discovered was that they should be integrated and that caring for both was what was needed to create a sense of peace and wholeness. Discovering this was what allowed Angela to love herself for the very first time.

Angela isn't the only one who came to us with an emotional eating habit. Renee, who arrived at the clinic at the age of forty-two, felt like food was her only comfort in life. She didn't care what she ate or how overeating might affect her health; food was her friend, and it was neither critical nor judgmental. She ate fatty foods without restriction, particularly indulging whenever she was stressed.

Renee had grown up feeling as if she was a disappointment to her parents. Throughout her life she worked tirelessly to please them, but they never gave her any positive attention. She was taught that she was disliked and unloved, and in turn, that's how she learned to treat herself as an adult. Her lack of self-respect landed her in a long and destructive relationship during which she was mistreated. Renee was hard on herself as well, always pursuing perfection to such an extent that she would essentially set herself up for failure.

As with Angela, Renee had to work to establish a Slimming Mindset before she could free herself from her emotional eating habit. She needed to look back at the responsibility and guilt she felt over not being able to please her parents and learn to let it go. This process allowed her to develop a new level of self-acceptance and eventually to love herself enough to take care of her body and health. A Slimming Mindset enabled her to automatically and reliably make better choices; instead of consistently engaging in habits that reflected a lack of self-respect, Renee learned to live a lifestyle that reflected the renewed sense of love she had for herself. This new way of living granted her weight loss and an incredible degree of self-confidence. She was truly transformed.

Do you see reflections of yourself in either Angela's or Renee's stories? Of course, your circumstances, experiences, and upbringing make your story unique, but if you see glimmers of yourself in some of their habits, it's important to ask yourself a few questions to see if you could be an emotional eater as well:

- Does your emotional state influence your eating habits?
- When you feel stressed, anxious, sad, or bored, do you turn to food for comfort?
- Do you eat as a response to physical hunger or emotional hunger?

Answering these questions honestly might take some time or require you to step back and analyze your habits a bit, especially since some emotional eating habits can be subconscious. Next time you have to deal with a stressful situation or strong emotions, pay attention to how you respond and what you reach for to soothe these feelings—if it's a bag of chips or a pint of ice cream, you'll find the exercises in the next section helpful in curbing your emotional eating habit.

The Importance of Self-Talk

If you've identified that you have emotional eating habits sabotaging your efforts to lose weight, we recommend you practice some mental exercises that will help you develop a new level of self-acceptance, a central element of creating a Slimming Mindset. When you operate from this mindset, you begin to make choices that reflect self-respect and not self-sabotage.

These exercises might sound a bit silly, but they can have a profound effect on your emotional well-being. We will be asking you to reflect on how you talk to yourself or, in other words, your self-talk. Whether you realize it or not, there is a constant dialogue going on in your head, and through this self-talk, you form a perception of yourself that has a significant impact on your happiness and well-being. How you talk to yourself not only determines how you feel each day but can also influence your health. A study published in the *Journal of the American Medical Association* found that a negative self-perception or severe lack of self-esteem is linked to a higher risk of illness and death.

The first step in the self-talk exercise is to begin to note how you talk to yourself throughout the day. Does your internal monologue have a cheerful and supportive tone, or is it critical and demeaning? The problem with negative self-talk is that it can be sneaky—it might be dominating the conversation in your head without you even realizing it, especially if it's been a practice of yours for some time. Can you recognize negative self-talk? Let's see what it might look like in a real-life scenario.

Suppose you're going to attend a social event, but your dress clothes no longer fit. So you decide to go shopping, but you're anxious about having to, once again, go through the painful experience of trying to find clothes that make you look good. When you arrive at the store and check out the racks, you find an outfit you like, but it turns out to be too small. The clerk brings you the next size up, but that one is still too small. Finally, you find a size that fits, but it looks shapeless and a bit bulky on you.

On the way home, you start talking to yourself, and the self-talk isn't good (think about what you might be saying in your own head in this scenario). Here are some of the thoughts that could be occurring:

I can't stand myself.

I'm disgusting.

I'm a total failure.

Who would ever want to be around me?

I can't go to this event.

I don't want to be seen in public.

I will never maintain a normal weight.

No matter what I do, I always gain weight.

Diets just don't work for me.

I'm hopeless.

These are thoughts that Renee or Angela and many of our participants might have running through their minds. The problem with this pessimistic self-talk is that it often gets stuck on repeat, and the more often you hear such statements, the more believable they become. Once negativity becomes part of your belief system, your behavior begins to confirm your thoughts. Then, negative thoughts become a habit and, once they're an automatic habit, they're extremely difficult to change. There's a point when negativity is so strong that it makes accepting, respecting, and loving yourself a monumental challenge. But don't worry; others have overcome this cycle of negativity and so can you.

There are two steps to improving your self-talk. First, you must take the power away from any negative thoughts you have in your head and remove them. Next, you must learn how to practice positive self-talk. Here's how it works:

STEP ONE: REMOVING NEGATIVE SELF-TALK

You've already started paying attention to your negative self-talk, but now we want you to document the dialogue. Take out a piece of paper or your journal and write out a list of your negative self-talk—don't rush; really take the time to connect with yourself and listen to the thoughts that spring from your head, or work to recall thoughts from past situations. This might feel uncomfortable at first, but it's the only way to understand and change negative thoughts.

Now, take a look at your list and analyze the statements. Read what you've written down and consider the strength and truth of the messages. When you really, truly pay attention to these thoughts, can you look at them and say they pass the truth test? Meaning, are they absolutely, 100 percent true? There are undoubtedly cracks in the logic—and when cracks are revealed, the whole system can crumble.

For example, let's look at the statement "I can't stand myself." This statement implies that you not only dislike yourself, but you dislike yourself so intensely that you can't live with it. At face value, that statement doesn't pass the truth test since you've probably learned to live with this feeling for a long time. Furthermore, there have undoubtedly been times when you didn't dislike yourself at all—in fact, if you think about it, there were certainly times when you actually liked yourself at least to some degree. So is that statement completely true? No.

Now we want you to write down a rational statement, one that will pass the truth test. This statement might be about your humiliating shopping experience (yes, this is hypothetical, but for the sake of this exercise, imagine it as your own or think about a similar experience in its place). Sure, you weren't happy with the experience or with yourself, but let's view the situation from another perspective. Instead of thinking about your reaction to the clothes not fitting, let's focus more on your feelings about your situation. A rational statement would be something more along the lines of "I feel terrible about not being able to manage my weight."

That statement passes the truth test, yet it's still incomplete. To complete the statement, we have to consider the other factors that may have contributed to your struggles with weight. Faulty information on nutrition, behaviors and eating patterns ingrained in you as a child, lack of trusted guidance—all of these can contribute to or perpetuate weight gain. Therefore, we could extend the statement to say, "I feel terrible about not being able to manage my weight—but considering all the faulty education and information I've been given all my life, my behavior is understandable."

If you compare the original self-talk statement to this more accurate final version, you can't help but feel better about yourself. Looking at the bigger, more complete picture allows you a certain freedom from sole responsibility, which can crush your self-esteem; you deserve to see the whole truth, and that means taking into consideration all the other influences that have shaped who you are today. This isn't about placing blame on other people or circumstances but rather about being kinder and gentler to yourself through a stronger connection with reality.

The goal for you now is to take this exercise and begin to apply it to your self-talk. Anytime you catch yourself thinking negatively about yourself, pause and consider if the statement running through your head passes the truth test. Then work to reconstruct the thought as we did in this exercise, taking your original shortsighted thought and transforming it to one that's more grounded, rational, and kind.

Remember, the negative thoughts have become almost automatic, so they won't go away on their own. But if you keep reshaping them from a rational perspective and repeating the new thoughts, these will eventually replace the irrational negative thoughts.

STEP TWO: PRACTICING POSITIVE SELF-TALK

Once you've learned to deal with your negative self-talk, you must work on replacing it with positive self-talk. We've discovered that an effective way to train yourself to self-talk positively is to think about the person you love most in your world—this could be a parent, a spouse, a friend, or anyone you respect. When you think about this person, try to analyze the ways in which you address them. Think about the tone you take with them and the language you use when you speak to them. It's probably a tone that's full of kindness and compassion, and ultimately love—the reason you use this tone with them is due to the love you feel for them. It's time to start reflecting on yourself from the same place of love and care.

You should treat yourself as you treat the person you love most in the world. If you address yourself with anything less than this level of consideration, catch yourself and work to redraft your thoughts. If it doesn't come easily at first, don't be concerned. You are likely working against years of negative self-perception and, in some cases, negativity that's been ingrained in you since you were a child. Be diligent and all-embracing with the love you direct your own way—there's no reason to hold back.

Visualizing Success

As much as your mind uses language to shape beliefs, it also uses imagery. We know that Angela saw herself as fat because her mother told her she was fat, and Renee saw herself as a hopeless failure because she never received any positive attention from her parents. Both of these women were practicing what's referred to as negative visualization.

Part of breaking free from a tendency to use food to soothe feelings is learning new strategies for creating and growing positive feelings. This can establish a more consistent emotional balance, which will help make you better equipped to deal with distressing emotions. We teach positive visualization as a way of boosting motivation and as a method for working through scenarios that might lead back to destructive eating habits; you're going to learn how to use it in both cases.

To practice positive visualization, it's essential to set aside fifteen minutes for yourself each day. And you will need to find a quiet place to get the most out of this exercise—try to go somewhere with few distractions—no telephones, dogs barking, or children demanding your attention. When you've found the right space, get comfortable and close your eyes. Take five slow and deep breaths, exhaling slower than inhaling.

For motivation: Visualize yourself in one month's time. See yourself stepping off the scale ecstatic about your progress. Imagine yourself walking into your closet, where you try on a favorite pair of pants you haven't fit into for years. You slip them on and, to your pleasant surprise, they fit great. Now, visualize yourself at the mirror taking it all in, noticing your face, belly, and hips and the changes you see—they've gotten thinner and smaller, and you see a healthy glow in your face. You might even give yourself a smile. This is you happy and successfully working toward your goal. Imagine how good this moment will feel for you.

Aim to do this visualization exercise each day for fourteen days. If you stick with it, you will find that your attitude and motivation will soar.

For dealing with distressing situations: Positive visualization is also an effective way to re-envision a circumstance that repeatedly leads to frustration for you. Let's use parents as the learning example since we often find that the dynamics involved are ripe with resentment and reflexive responses. In this example, imagine yourself having followed the Love Diet for five or six weeks. You're feeling great about your progress, and you've proudly established some healthy new eating habits. And then your mom invites you to dinner. You know how your mom does dinner—if there are eight people invited for dinner, she'll cook for eighteen. On top of that, vegetables rarely land on the dinner table, and if they do, they're covered in cheese, butter, or mayo. Plus, she'll push the breadbasket like her life depended on it: "You *have* to eat some bread!" What's worse is that this is the food you were raised on, your personal soul food. How do you head to dinner and make sure you both enjoy it and emerge without having sabotaged all your hard work?

You make a visit ahead of time to your quiet space for fifteen minutes of visualization. Once there, complete the same breathing exercises as before and get into the mental space to practice visualization. Visualize yourself driving up to Mom's house. You walk in the front door and smell the aroma of her cooking. You take in the scents and sights of home, and you see everyone getting ready to have dinner. But you see things happening differently this time, perhaps for the first time.

Visualize yourself unwrapping the dish that you brought for your dinner—it's a dish that is healthful and on your plan. You sit at the table with your healthful food and watch the others ignoring your dish while they're loading up on excessive amounts of carbohydrates. You're enjoying your meal and the conversation when you find yourself flashing back to that frustrating trip to the store you took a few weeks ago. You remember the outfit you wanted, the frustration you felt when it was two sizes too small, and the negative cycle of emotions sparked by that experience. Then, see yourself looking back at all the carbohydrate-heavy foods and realizing that if you continue to eat those foods, you're going to need larger clothes, not smaller clothes, and you're going to get more bad news at the doctor's office instead of the good news you've been waiting for. You smile and take another bite of your healthy dinner. On your way home, you feel like you've just climbed the highest mountain, and you feel terrific and thrilled by your accomplishment.

Visualization is a powerful tool. If you first create a new reality in your mind, you can then live it in your life. If you practice it, along with the positive self-talk techniques, you will find that you start to feel more in control of your life. You'll begin to move away from obsessive approaches to dieting and toward healthy eating strategies. It won't feel difficult to implement these strategies; they'll seem like a natural part of taking care of yourself. You will feel an unprecedented sort of balance in your emotions and your overall approach to life. Your stress, brain fog, anger, mood swings, agitated mind, and sleep problems will lessen, and you won't feel the need to turn to food for help. Instead, you will turn to a much more powerful tool: your mind, which you now know how to use to manifest a better destiny and visualize a brighter future.

How You Eat: Are You a Mindless Eater?

Mindless eating is a form of almost subconscious eating; it happens when you eat and overeat without paying attention, or when you find yourself consuming something simply out of habit.

If you've ever eaten an entire bag of chips while watching TV, you've engaged in mindless eating. If you've gone through a whole package of cookies while working away on the computer, you've practiced mindless eating. If the aroma of Cinnabon at the mall has drawn you in to pick up cinnamon rolls (and you weren't even hungry), you've given in to mindless eating. (In this latter case, the mindless part is more about the habit cue and your response—more on this later.) This type of eating, which involves a zombielike tuning out, almost always correlates to overeating. The good news is that with some careful attention to your daily habits, you can eliminate mindless eating impulses entirely.

Habits are difficult to form, but they're even harder to change or eliminate, and for good reason—habits are useful. Imagine driving down the road and being occupied with whether to use your right foot on the brake, then wondering how hard to press the pedal, and when to start pressing that pedal every time you intend to stop. It would be like learning to drive each time you got into your car. Habits make this relearning experience unnecessary.

In routine situations, habits trigger action hundreds if not thousands of times a day. You can zip up a zipper or take a sip of water or brush your teeth without taxing your brain to any significant extent; your habits have taught you how to do these things without paying too much attention. In this way, you are able to save your brainpower for novel or creative tasks—it's really a matter of resource conservation. Without this storage ability, humans would be highly inefficient and could not have evolved as they have.

Of course, not all habits are useful. Eating chips while watching TV, bingeing on beer at the ball game, or stopping at the Starbucks on the way home for a double Frappuccino aren't constructive habits. In fact, they're more likely to be destructive when it comes to your health and weight.

Habits are created by behavior repetition, and once created, habits usually remain automatic. They occur in a cycle that begins with a cue and results in an action. A cue alerts your mind that a certain behavior should be performed in response to a stimulus (these patterns are stored in your brain). For example, in the case of being drawn into the bakery at the mall, the bakery's aroma is the cue, and the behavioral action that follows—eating the cinnamon roll—can become a habit. When the action triggers temporary feelings of pleasure through a reward center response, as sugary, highly processed snacks and drinks do, the habit will then be reinforced and inevitably grow stronger. As a habit gains strength your sensitivity to the cue increases and the behavior pattern becomes increasingly automatic. And before you know it, every time you're at the mall, it happens like clockwork: you smell the cinnamon rolls and then you stop to eat one. It's officially become a habit. You can see how it works in this graphic:

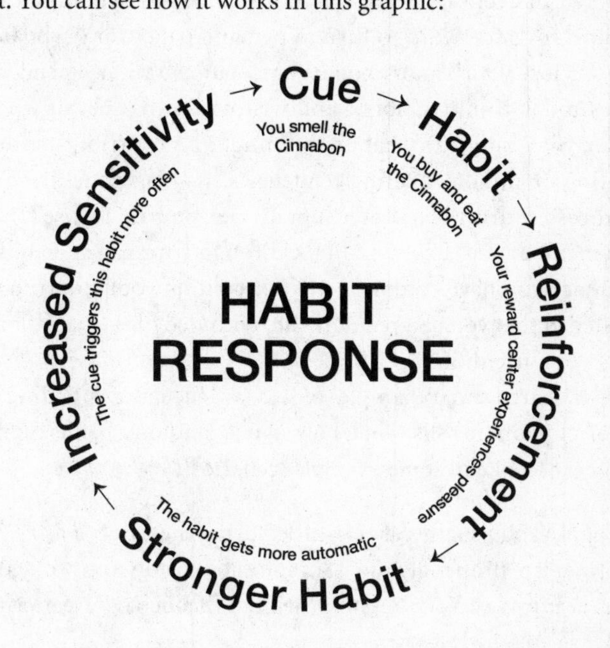

The problem with this cycle of behavior is that you begin to do things without conscious thought or authentic desire. And the more you repeat this pattern, the stronger the habit gets, which makes it more difficult to break.

Many different types of stimuli can act as cues. Your senses of smell, taste, sight, or sound can cue a habit; so can the time of day, holidays, locations, people, and emotions. Our most powerful habits are called keystone habits, in reference to the center stone of an ancient Roman arch that kept the arch suspended. And like the stone that centrally supported the arch, every person has keystone habits that support other habit groups. When you change your keystone habits, others change automatically.

It's important to identify your unhealthy habits, especially your keystone habits, and the cues that trigger them. Habits can be difficult to identify because they're so much a part of your pattern that it's easy to overlook them.

To get an accurate grasp on your habits—the good and bad—it's important once again to turn to pen and paper (or keyboard and screen, or just your smartphone) for documentation. Spend fifteen minutes today thinking about and writing down a list of what you consider your unhealthy habits that might be contributing to your overeating or mindless eating tendencies. If this seems like a difficult process, enlist the aid of a support person like a close friend or family member—sit down and talk through your eating habits with them. Once you have compiled a list, keep it on your smartphone or computer so that you can regularly be reminded of the habits most in need of your attention.

We've shared some examples of habits—such as responding to the smell of cinnamon rolls—but how about keystone habits? Let's see what they look like in some example scenarios.

- Suppose you usually eat very little during the day, but after your normal late dinner at 8:00 P.M., you eat nonstop until you go to bed at 1:00 A.M. Your keystone habit in that behavior pattern is your sleep schedule.
- Another example is snacking while watching TV. The keystone habit in this case is TV watching.

In both cases, the habits of overeating or mindless eating will be broken if you change the keystone habit. In the first instance, altering your sleep time (see tips on how to do this in the Resources section) and going to bed earlier will break up the nighttime binge habit. In the second example, you might try finding alternative forms of entertainment until you break the habit or only watch TV with a group of people who don't mindlessly snack.

Take a moment to examine your habit list to see if you can identify the keystone habits that might have triggered the type of destructive habits that can lead to weight gain. One way to deal with these habits is to remove the cues from your environment; in other words, to remove the first domino that sets the habit response in motion. Don't drive home past your favorite Frappuccino shop, don't eat at the restaurant where you normally overeat, don't keep junk food in the house, and so on. Develop a plan to modify these habits. Then get your support people to assist you in making changes, but also be aware that habits can take a considerable time to change fully.

Beyond Emotional and Mindless Eating: Beware When Too Much Is Never Enough

While most of the people who visit our clinic demonstrate emotional eating or mindless eating habits, there are others who have a more complicated relationship with food due to a binge-eating disorder. Binge eating is not uncommon among people who struggle with weight; in fact, statistics show that 30 percent of people who enter any diet program are binge eaters. Bingeing is different from emotional eating, mindless eating, or just ordinary overeating. While there is some overlap between all three, if you are a binge eater, you are likely to feel completely out of control of how much food you eat, and you may even describe eating as a sort of out-of-body experience.

It's impossible to create permanent weight loss if an underlying binge-eating disorder isn't addressed and treated. Most binge eaters will rapidly gain weight back once an eating program is ended, and they're more likely to become morbidly obese, which can be truly life threatening.

If you think you might have binge-eating tendencies, you should take it very seriously. Following are some questions to help identify if you're a binge eater or not as well as some suggestions for dealing with the disorder. If you find that even after trying some of the strategies, you're still struggling with binge eating, be sure to seek additional help from a psychologist or counselor who is experienced in dealing with binge-eating disorders.

Are You a Binge Eater?

Answer these questions to see if your habits might suggest a binge-eating disorder:

- Do you engage in rapid eating? Answer yes if you eat so fast that there's a lag between eating and your feelings of fullness or overfullness.
- Do you eat to a point of discomfort? Answer yes if you often feel noticeably uncomfortable after a meal, to the point that your fullness interferes with movement, sleeping, or any other part of your normal routine.
- Do you eat when you're not hungry? Answer yes if you eat again soon after you've eaten a full meal or when you're not hungry, or if you regularly go back for seconds and thirds.
- Do you hide your eating? Answer yes if you hide the type or quantity of food you eat from others, and if you conceal evidence of your eating.
- Do you eat alone so you won't be judged? Answer yes if you prefer to eat alone so you can eat as much as you want and whatever you want without embarrassment. This might include avoiding social situations where eating is involved.
- Do you feel out of control with your eating? Answer yes if you feel that you should stop eating but cannot, or if you make promises to yourself or others about your eating and then quickly break them.
- Do you feel guilt, shame, or disgust about your eating? Answer yes if you wake up disgusted with yourself over your eating, or if you feel ashamed of what you ate or how much you ate.
- Do you wake up in the middle of the night to eat? Answer yes if you engage in midnight meals or if you eat most of your daily calories after dinner.

You may have a binge-eating problem if you answered yes to three or more of these questions, you feel this way at least twice a week, and it's been going on for at least six months. Keep in mind that this isn't by any means a clinical diagnosis, but if you meet the criteria, you could benefit greatly from following these suggestions as you begin the Seven Stages (the diet portion of *The Love Diet*):

- **Do not hide your food or your eating:** This is a red flag warning of the return of a binge-eating disorder. Make an effort to eat with other people to keep yourself from secretive eating habits.
- **Do not eat after dinner:** There is a very high rate of association between night-eating syndrome and a binge-eating disorder. Be sure to eat meals and snacks during the day so you don't get over-hungry at night.
- **Track, track, . . . and track!** Write down everything that goes into your mouth within fifteen minutes of eating. Doing it at the end of the day or tomorrow or next week does not work if you're a binge eater. Meal tracking is the best way not only to track your eating behavior but also to keep it under control.
- **Do not base your feelings of success or failure on the scale:** The scale is a lagging indicator. That means you can be well into your disordered eating before the scale starts to move, and that could be too late. The best indicator of success or failure is your meal tracker. It is real-time and can alert you to problems immediately.
- **Become a regular and consistent exerciser:** A consistent exercise habit has proven to help binge eaters maintain control. Getting a workout buddy can help ensure accountability and get you out the door when you're feeling less motivated. You might even consider finding a backup workout buddy who you can reach out to when your regular workout partner is sick, out of town, or otherwise unavailable.
- **Surround yourself with supporters:** The more open you are about your commitment to better your eating habits, the more likely you are to stick with it. Share your goals with your spouse, significant other, or good friends, and consider asking one of them to be your support contact. You don't have to ask them to help hold you

accountable (although you can)—just sharing your plans with them will help shore up your own commitment to yourself.

- **Love yourself!** You can't get better if you spend time beating yourself up or thinking negative thoughts. Remember that the Slimming Mindset is a vital part of success on the Seven Stages, and that means learning how to accept, respect, and love yourself (see page 18 for more). You must love yourself even through lapses, and you must be encouraging with your self-talk.
- **Stay on Stage 2 of the Seven Stages:** If you find that you're struggling with binge eating while following the program, return to Stage 2 and stay there until you have reached your goal weight. Then gradually transition carefully through the remaining stages. Sticking to just this one part of the eating plan may help build your confidence and leave less room for slipups.

The One-Size-Fits-All Solution to Overeating

In this chapter, we've shared with you specific strategies that will help you if you're a mindless eater, an emotional eater, or a binge eater. But no matter what compels you to overeat, whether it's habits, emotions, or a genetic disposition, there is one factor that needs to be the central element of your plan to break up with overeating: love. Throughout the program, it's essential that you make a standing commitment to check in with love, particularly as it relates to your eating habits. If you catch yourself falling off track or eating in a way that won't help you achieve your weight loss or health goals, pause and ask yourself if what you're doing reflects your promise to love, accept, and respect yourself and your body. If the answer is no, put an end to the activity and move on with your day.

PART II

Getting Ready to Change Your Life

CHAPTER 4

The Five Core Concepts

Whenever you start an eating or exercise program, or take on any endeavor new to you, usually what follows is a series of *whys*: "Why am I doing this? Why am I doing that?" And we have found in our experience that, when it comes to weight loss, when a person can't answer *why*, a door is opened to an excuse. To help make sure that door is never opened for you, we're addressing here some of the most commonly asked *whys* we encounter as people begin the Seven Stages. The answers will introduce you to five core concepts that together form the nutritional foundation of the Seven Stages. Think of these as trusted diet lessons that will help deepen your commitment through greater understanding.

1. Why We Eliminate Sugar and Simple Carbs

Understanding how different foods impact your blood sugar is one of the most important steps toward taking control of your weight—it can truly be a life-changing understanding if it translates to real changes in how you eat. Since sugar and simple carbohydrates have the most significant impact on your blood sugar, it's essential to learn a bit about how they affect your body.

Let's first establish some basics on carbohydrates. There are two types of carbs: simple and complex. Simple carbohydrates are any sugar-containing foods like fruit, candy, and cookies and sweetened beverages such as soda and fruit juice. Your body burns these rapidly so they are great for a quick burst of energy, but they do not satisfy your appetite. They also can cause a rapid spike in blood sugar followed by a significant drop, which puts you on a carb-craving roller coaster. Complex carbohydrates include starchy and nonstarchy vegetables, legumes, and whole grains. Complex carbohydrates that are rich in fiber and healthful nutrients don't result in a rapid spike and allow for a slower drop in blood sugar, minimizing extreme hunger or fatigue. After Stage 1, nonstarchy vegetables will be your go-to complex carbohydrate. They're relatively low in carbohydrates and rich in fiber and nutrients, making them both filling and good for you.

When compared to the other macronutrients—protein and fat—both forms of carbohydrates create a more significant response in your blood sugar. However, this chart will help you see the drastic difference between simple carbohydrates and the other individual macronutrients.

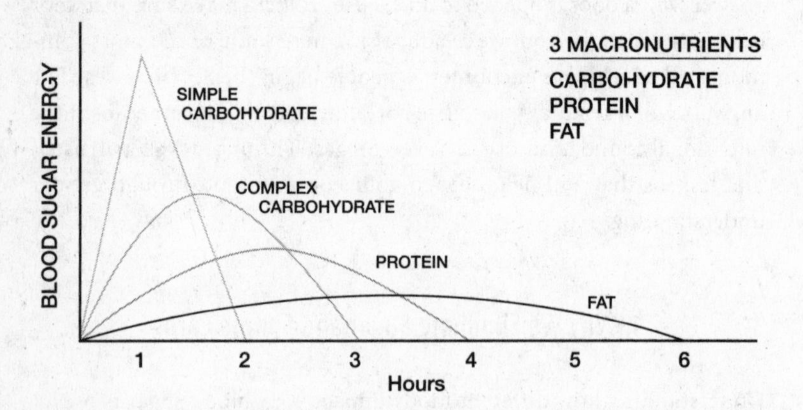

You can see that the blood sugar response to simple carbohydrates is extreme when compared to other macronutrients. What happens during (and after) this surge is a series of events that sets you up for weight gain. The spike in blood sugar can activate your reward center, which—as noted in the previous chapter—establishes a dangerous association between certain foods and feeling good. A rapid drop in blood sugar will follow the surge and stimulate hunger—and not just any hunger, but the intense, carb-craving, I'm-going-to-eat-an-entire-bag-of-chips kind of hunger. The drop in blood sugar is so extreme that, after you've eaten simple carbohydrates, you are practically programmed to reach for more of the same thing, because declining blood sugar signals to the body that it's in need of some fast-acting foods, i.e., more sugar.

By comparison, complex carbohydrates produce a much more moderate blood sugar response. Complex carbohydrates contain fiber, which helps slow digestion, leading to a gradual rise in blood sugar levels. Proteins and fats trigger an even lower blood sugar response, with the flatter curves representing the more stable blood sugar response. Foods that produce a lower measured response of blood sugar create greater satiety and help stave off hunger for longer periods of time.

The consequence of getting an increasing number of your calories from simple carbohydrates, such as sugar, is often the development of a layer of body fat around your waist. You might refer to this type of body fat as just belly fat, but it also has a clinical name: central adipose tissue. No matter what you call it, it can be especially damaging. Central adipose tissue can cause the body to produce inflammatory chemicals that negatively affect many of the body's systems. It also can lead to insulin resistance, meaning that insulin begins to lose its ability to help move the sugar in your blood into the cells where it is needed. The result of this process is often type 2 diabetes.

Why should you be concerned? If you have diabetes, you are two to five times more likely to have coronary artery disease and heart attacks. Forty-four percent of people with diabetes will develop atherosclerosis, and 25 percent will develop kidney disease. In fact, if your blood sugar level is frequently above normal, you are almost guaranteed to be at risk for health complications related to inflammation.

Regaining control of your blood sugar begins with eliminating sugar and starchy carbs from your diet. The average person today consumes over 150 pounds of sugar a year—that's over 16,000 teaspoons of sugar! The acceptable amount of added sugar is 6 teaspoons per day for women (20 pounds per year) and 9 teaspoons per day for men (30 pounds per year). It's impossible to lose weight or even maintain a healthy weight when sugar intake is as high as it is in an average person's diet. One of the quickest ways to cut sugar is to remove sugar-sweetened beverages, like soft drinks, from your diet. Believe it or not, a single can of soda contains the equivalent of 8.25 teaspoons of sugar,

WHAT ABOUT HIGH FRUCTOSE CORN SYRUP?

Among a growing number of health practitioners, there's increased awareness that consuming excessive amounts of high fructose corn syrup (HFCS) has a negative effect on health. HFCS rapidly enters your bloodstream and goes directly to your liver, where it is made into fat and increases the blood levels of cholesterol and triglycerides. Research shows that high intake of HFCS can also lead to an increase in weight as well as the risk for a fatty liver, which can lead to cirrhosis, liver cancer, liver failure, and death.

while a 32-ounce cup of sports drink, soda, or sweetened tea can contain up to 21 teaspoons!

Refined carbohydrates, such as white bread, white rice, and white pasta, aren't any better for you. These foods deliver few nutrients and yet are high in the type of calories that will quickly be stored as body fat. This is why a large plate of white rice or white pasta or a giant bowl of cereal won't keep you full for a prolonged period. Over time, excessive intake of refined carbs leads to an increased risk of inflammation, heart disease, and diabetes.

All forms of sugar, including simple and refined carbohydrates, will cause weight gain and lead to blood sugar imbalances that impact your appetite control, mood, and energy level. Research has also linked excess consumption of these types of foods to other health issues and complications, including:

- Visceral adiposity, the very dangerous buildup of fat in your abdominal region that is linked to metabolic syndrome, heart disease, stroke, and cancer
- Suppression of your immune system
- Increased inflammatory response in your entire body
- A rise in fat levels circulating in your blood, leading to atherosclerosis (plaque buildup in the arteries)
- Damage to your kidneys and liver

ARE YOU IMBALANCED?

If you have been a yo-yo dieter for years and put your body through a rotation of extreme dieting to binge eating and back again, you are most likely out of biochemical balance. Symptoms of imbalance include frequent and extreme cravings—especially for carbohydrates—fatigue, dizziness, mood swings, and energy dips. Most of our participants at 20/20 LifeStyles come to us with symptoms of imbalance. And tests usually confirm that 1) their response to insulin and carbs is blunted, meaning they've stopped using foods for energy in an efficient manner, and 2) they have borderline high blood sugar levels. If you've experienced symptoms of imbalance, it's likely that you have these underlying metabolic issues as well. Stage 1 will focus directly on restoring blood sugar balance and improving insulin response, allowing you to experience quick and noticeable results, especially in "waist" loss. You'll immediately start to feel more energy and more in control of your cravings for sweets and carbs.

- Damage to your arteries and heart
- Stomach problems
- Vision problems

Given all the evidence, it's easy to see why the first step in the Seven Stages is to remove sugar and simple carbohydrates from your diet. When you eliminate these, you restore metabolic balance and open the door to steady, reliable weight loss.

2. Why Grains Have to Go (At Least for a Little While)

While there is a general consensus that true whole grains offer protective health benefits, most so-called healthful foods containing grains aren't so healthy after all. They're more likely to be processed, refined grains with misleading labels: phrases like *100% wheat, multigrain,* or *cracked wheat,* which have nothing to do with whether the bread or cereal is whole grain. Chances are, what you're really eating is refined grains that will quickly be broken down and stored as fat. A true whole grain food will have a *100% Whole Grain* label on its packaging, and the grain listed on an ingredient list should be identified as *whole* (you'll find more whole grain buying tips in Chapter 12).

At 20/20 LifeStyles, we've found that grains present digestive problems, rashes, cramping, and irritable bowel syndrome and contribute to feelings of low energy and difficulty concentrating. While the level of tolerance and sensitivity to grain products varies greatly by individual, a large percentage of people find that grains prevent weight loss or produce bloating or digestive discomfort. This is why it's especially important to document any responses you have to grains when they're added back into your diet during Stage 7. If you notice that your progress slows or you develop symptoms of discomfort, you might find that, like Kim, you want to remove grains from your diet for good.

When Kim came to us, we discovered that she, like many others, had grown up in a culture where good behavior was rewarded with food. She also learned to view food as love from a very young age; when her dad passed away when she was eight, her mom regularly tried to console Kim's grief with food.

Kim carried these associations with food into adulthood, when she found herself using food to deal with almost any emotion. By the time she was fifty-two, she realized that food had become a crutch and she relied on it completely with no regard for what it was doing to her body.

Like many women nearing middle age, Kim pushed her weight and her health to a breaking point. She knew she needed help to take back control of her health. And this is where the Seven Stages came in. When Kim learned how to transform her diet and exercise habits, her entire life changed. She lost more than twenty pounds, developed renewed muscle tone, and felt fitter than she ever had in her life.

Looking back, Kim says she's amazed to have been so unaware of her unhealthy eating habits. She really had no awareness of the damage she was doing to her body each and every day through her diet.

Like millions of other people, Kim used to eat all kinds of grain-based products without giving it a thought. Pizza, pasta, bread, cereals, and crackers were a major part of her diet. She had never considered how these types of foods were affecting her body. It wasn't until she removed grains during the Seven Stages that she noticed the difference. Without grains, she started to feel more energetic, and her mental fogginess and uncontrollable cravings were eliminated. It wasn't until she added them back in during Stage 7 that she fully understood that grains weren't good for her body and decided to eliminate them for good.

Kim became living proof that the elimination of grains from a regular diet works. She enthusiastically tells others that her body feels so much better now that she's off a high-grain diet. During the program, she eliminated grains for almost two months as she was working through the other stages. While she was accustomed to having breads, cereals, and pasta as part of her meals—as most of us are—she found removing them made room for so many other delicious and filling foods. Kim enjoyed eating more lean protein–rich meals with chicken, seafood, and beef, and getting all of the complex carbohydrates she needed from colorful vegetables, which are rich in protective antioxidants, vitamins, and minerals.

Eventually, she was able to transition to limited use of whole grains, but even then she realized she had felt so much better without them. Kim decided to keep grains out of her diet for good, and even her family has learned to adapt to this change. Her husband and kids eat more fruit, vegetables, and lean protein, and they look forward to finding delicious new ways to prepare fresh salads and vegetables. Sandwiches are now made with lettuce wraps, and pasta dishes and pizzas are no longer on the menu. Kim and her family are in better health for it.

3. Why We Focus on Protein and Vegetables

Protein and vegetables will become mainstays on your plate throughout the Seven Stages (and beyond if you'd like to maintain a healthy weight). If simple and refined carbs create intense cravings and low energy and program your body to store fat, protein and nonstarchy vegetables could be said to do the opposite. Foods with protein, such as eggs, chicken, fish, lean meats, and tofu, keep you fuller longer and help your body repair itself. Protein is made up of amino acids, which are the building materials of skin, muscle, bone, and even enzymes and hormones that you need for digestion, metabolism, and other important functions.

The other benefit of eating foods rich in lean protein is their effect on insulin, which if you remember the graph from earlier in the chapter, is very little. When you keep insulin low, you will prevent continuous fat storage (i.e., weight gain) from occurring. Of course, this is only true if you eat the right quality of proteins. Hot dogs might have protein, but they are also full of additives and saturated fat that can impact your weight and long-term health. You'll discover all the best sources of protein when you start following the Seven Stages in Chapter 6.

As for vegetables, everyone knows they're good for you. What people don't always know is how filling and versatile vegetables can be—they are essential to creating meals that satisfy hunger *and* make you feel good.

At 20/20 LifeStyles, we work hard to create vegetable lovers out of everyone who enters the program. And to tell you the truth, it will be easier to fall in love with vegetables once you've begun to work your way through the Seven Stages. When you reset your body during the first stage, you transform your taste buds to some degree. Years of overindulgence in sweet, fatty, and salty foods can desensitize your taste buds to the point that natural flavors don't satisfy. However, after just a short period of eating simple, fresh foods your taste buds will come back to life and you'll be amazed at the punch of flavor natural foods offer. Nonstarchy vegetables that you never thought you liked will suddenly be appealing. Always been an asparagus hater? Try it in our Grilled Asparagus Salad recipe after you've reached Stage 3 of the plan.

Of course, we can't talk about vegetables without acknowledging their many incredible health benefits. Consuming multiple servings of vegetables a day has been linked to reduced risk of most chronic diseases including heart disease, diabetes, and obesity. The simplest and most powerful thing you can do to improve your health is to eat more colorful vegetables. They are rich in vitamins, minerals, and nutrients that can help lower stress, improve eyesight, increase energy, accelerate weight loss, boost your mood, and improve circulation, bone health, and skin. Oh, and did we mention they're low in fat and calories too?

VEGGIE POWER: MORE BENEFITS THAN YOU CAN COUNT

If vegetables came with labels listing their benefits like packaged foods list their ingredients, most veggies would have to grow a great deal bigger—there are just too many to list! Increasing your overall vegetable consumption is one of the simplest ways to improve your overall health. Vegetables can:

- Decrease your risk for stroke and heart attack
- Protect against several types of cancers
- Lower blood pressure
- Improve digestion
- Guard against cataracts
- Save your memory as you get older
- Help you lose weight by providing maximum nutrients at minimum calories

You don't have to wait until you begin the Seven Stages to start eating more vegetables—spend more time in the produce aisle today and bring some good health home. Start stocking up!

4. Why Alcohol Is the Diet Destroyer

Our recommendation on alcohol is one of the most impactful changes we've made to the eating plan over the years. Initially, we allowed program participants to have one glass of wine per week. The calories in one glass of wine—about 120—seemed insignificant enough that over the course of just one week, it would not have an impact on progress or results. That ended up not being the case. We found that even just one glass of wine would lead to less weight loss or no weight loss at all during that week. It had to be more than the calories.

Further research revealed that it has to do with how the body responds to alcohol. When alcohol hits your system, a compound is created that gives your body a signal that it's in a high-energy state, meaning there's an abundance of fuel in your system. This compound is created regardless of the calories in the alcoholic beverage you've had, and it essentially switches your body to the metabolic processes that are associated with storing energy, otherwise known as fat production. When energy is stored instead of burned, this puts the brakes on weight loss and accelerates weight gain.

Additionally, alcohol is empty calories—it contains no nutritional value. Alcohol is also a disinhibitor, which means it negatively affects your judgment and can make it tough to stick to your goals to eat well. You might be able to say no to a late-night plate of nachos if you haven't been drinking, but add a few drinks to the equation and you'll likely be indulging in sabotage snacking.

We will address how to add alcohol back into your diet later in the maintenance chapter. If you find it difficult to cut out alcohol during the Seven Stages, it might be time to evaluate your relationship with alcohol. Just remember that everything we advise you to do during this program has a specific, unified purpose, and that is to help you lose weight and regain your health. If the thought of giving up alcohol or anything else during the Seven Stages creates stress or anxiety in you, we recommend trying to shift your mindset—don't focus on what you might be giving up, but instead look at what you will be gaining.

5. Why We Teach that There's No Such Thing as "Free" Foods

Foods are often advertised as being free of fat, sugar, and, with increasing popularity, gluten. The problem with these "fat-free," "sugar-free," and "gluten-free" foods is that many people mistakenly believe that these labels are synonymous with a food being healthful—and that's far from the truth. Consumers like you aren't the ones to blame—it's the companies that jump on the bandwagon to sell more of their products. While they may not explicitly say on their packaging that a certain food is healthful, they know the right labels will make you *think* something is healthful.

Sugar-free foods became popular as more and more people began seeking foods that were diabetic friendly. Instead of sweetening with cane or beet sugars or high fructose corn syrup, companies began sweetening foods and drinks with artificial sweeteners such as aspartame, saccharin, stevia, and sucralose. While the FDA claims that these substances are safe, groups such as the American Heart Association and the American Diabetes Association suggest careful use of them. There is research that suggests artificial sweeteners can lead to weight gain and modify the balance of bacteria in your gut (which can impact weight, digestion, and your immune system). Oftentimes we find that people tend to overeat sugar-free foods because they've convinced themselves that sugar-free means calorie-free, which isn't the case. They also leave room for later indulgences—"I had a sugar-free diet soda with lunch, so I can eat a bunch of cookies tonight." Making rationalizations like this ultimately leads to greater calorie intake and eventual weight gain.

A fat-free craze swept this country in the late eighties after reports came out suggesting that limiting fat was the most important thing you could do for your health. And soon after, everybody's favorite foods were made available in low-fat or fat-free varieties. You could get fat-free cookies, tortillas and bread, and even fat-free milk, butter substitutes, and cheese. Everyone rushed to buy up all these new products to cut the fat from their diets.

What's wrong with fat-free foods? When fat is cut from foods, the flavor has to come from somewhere else, and more often than not, this somewhere is sugar. The problem with sugar being used as the replacement is that now the food will have a significant impact on your blood sugar and insulin, which you now know leads to greater fat storage and loss of appetite control. The use of sugar also doesn't change the calorie content all that much, despite the perception that low-fat and fat-free foods are better for weight loss. The movement away from fat pushed us toward eating more carbohydrates than ever and is likely a significant contributor to the unprecedented rise in weight gain and diseases of obesity such as type 2 diabetes and metabolic syndrome.

Gluten-free is the biggest and newest trend to hit the diet world in quite some time. Many people have begun to eliminate gluten from their diets based on the suggestion that foods containing gluten can cause weight gain, bloating, digestive discomfort, or a more serious allergic response. A true allergy to gluten is only seen in people with celiac disease, which affects about 1 percent of the population.

GET TO KNOW GLUTEN

You can't go too far these days in a grocery store without seeing the words *gluten-free* on a food's packaging. But unless you have celiac disease or know someone who does, you might not even know what gluten is. Gluten refers to the proteins found in wheat, which includes barley, rye, and triticale. You're probably not surprised to hear it can be found in breads, baked goods, cereals, and certain beers, but did you know that gluten is also used in soups, sauces, salad dressings, and spice mixes? It's used in these foods as an emulsifier, which binds ingredients together, enhancing a product's thickness.

For some people, eating gluten can be a real headache (literally). If you are intolerant to gluten, you might experience headaches, an upset stomach or abdominal pain, a foggy mind, or joint pain after you eat foods containing gluten. If you experience any of these symptoms up to two to three hours later, you might want to consider eliminating gluten for a period of time to see if the symptoms subside. (Although the Love Diet does eliminate grains through Stage 6, it is not a gluten-free eating plan).

As we discussed earlier, we eliminate grains (some of which contain gluten) from the first several stages of the Seven Stages. Many people experience surprising benefits from this elimination. They might feel more energetic or less bloated or deal with fewer digestive issues when grains are gone. Others find that grains and gluten don't bother them, but they might slow progress with weight loss. It all depends on the individual.

When it comes to gluten-free foods, the same issue exists here as with all other "free" foods—there is not necessarily a larger health benefit to eating them (unless you have a sensitivity to gluten). Many processed foods do not contain gluten. Sugar, high fructose corn syrup, and canola oil are all gluten-free. A Snickers candy bar is gluten-free, but that certainly doesn't mean it's healthy.

The bigger point here is that "free" foods all come at a price. It's important to question labels and not fall for something that seems too good to be true. In *The Love Diet,* we'll guide you toward a diet filled with foods you can trust and those that will help restore your health and not take it away. With that in mind, let's get to a preview of the Seven Stages.

The Seven Stages: At a Glance

When you get to the Seven Stages in the next part of the book, you'll see the five core concepts incorporated throughout. We emphasize reduced consumption of simple carbs, increased intake of lean proteins and vegetables, cutting out alcohol, and so on—but these aren't the only dietary principles informing the structure and strategy you'll see in the eating plan. In fact, every element has been carefully developed based on cutting-edge science in nutrition and weight management. Each detail of the eating plan has been tested and retested to ensure that it's ready to guide you through your journey to permanent weight loss and improved health. Here's how the stages will work:

Stage 1: Detox

In this stage you will eat only lean protein, berries, and some healthy fats. Berries will provide the carbohydrates you need without causing you to experience hunger or cravings. You will stay on this stage only one week to allow your body to detoxify and your metabolism to become balanced. The meals and foods eaten during this week will restore blood sugar balance and begin to transition your body from fat storing to fat burning.

Stage 2: Veggie Boost

Stage 2 will bring a burst of flavor, color, and texture. During this stage, you'll add back in nonstarchy vegetables. These are vegetables such as leafy greens, green beans, asparagus, broccoli, carrots, beets, cauliflower, and more. Many of you may choose to stay on this stage for up to two weeks. Stage 2 is your safe zone, where weight loss is rapid and hunger and cravings are absent. This is also a stage that you can return to if you find your progress slowing or hunger returning at any point in the later stages.

Stage 3: Protein Power

In this stage, we will add back in some higher-protein dairy-based foods such as low-fat cheese, low-fat or nonfat cottage cheese, and nonfat plain Greek yogurt. These foods will contribute to your daily protein requirements but will not replace your lean protein servings at meals. This will increase the number of foods you can eat to satisfy your protein requirements throughout the day. Remember, foods high in protein will help keep you fuller longer. You will feel satisfied and continue to maintain optimal metabolic functions—this means your body will stay in a fat-burning zone!

Stage 4: Favorite Fruits

In Stage 4, you will get to reintroduce all fruits to your diet. We categorize berries as their own food group because they're higher in fiber and lower in sugar than all other fruits. The key to this stage is portion control. While you will continue to be able to consume one cup of berries, all other fruits will be limited to half a cup. This is because fruits are simple carbohydrates that, despite being full of vitamins and minerals, will be absorbed by your body very quickly. Fruit is an excellent source of quick energy, but it won't keep you satiated for a prolonged period of time.

Stage 5: Dairy Delights

In Stage 5, you will add back in all dairy, including fruit-flavored yogurts and milk. Dairy can produce digestive problems, increase hunger or cravings, or slow or stop weight loss, so it's important to pay attention to how your body feels during this stage. If you notice any negative effects caused by particular foods, you can simply remove those again and monitor how you feel.

Stage 6: Legume Love

In Stage 6, you will reintroduce legumes to your diet. This includes beans, lentils, and split peas. Beans are the most commonly consumed food in the legume family and contain a small amount of protein. But since beans actually have two to three times more carbohydrate content than protein content, they are considered a carbohydrate. You can enjoy foods like chili, hummus (great for snacks!), and any of your favorite beans, such as kidney, black, or pinto, during this stage. We'll include suggestions on how to reduce the amount of sodium in the beans you buy (this will reduce bloating and water retention).

Stage 7: Grains and Starchy Vegetables

This is the final stage of the plan. At this point, all food groups will have been reintroduced into your diet. You'll be able to eat whole grains again, which will include everything from bread, rice, pasta, and cereal to snack foods like pretzels and crackers. And starchy vegetables will be on the menu again too. This includes foods such as corn, peas, potatoes, sweet potatoes, and winter squash.

As with others who've come to us at 20/20 LifeStyles, you might find that with the return of grain-based foods comes the return of your overeating habits or digestive problems. It's within your power—and perfectly healthy—to remove them again. Grains are not necessary for optimal health, and many people find their health and weight are much better off without grains in their diets. After you complete all seven stages, it will be up to you to identify what works best for you.

In Part III, you'll take the first steps toward permanent weight loss when you begin Stage 1, but before you do that, be sure to check out the next chapter to make sure you have everything you need to succeed on the plan.

CHAPTER 5

Before You Begin: Habits, Tips, and Tools to Help Make the Love Diet Your Last Diet

Success doesn't just happen—you have to make it happen—and a big part of making success happen is ensuring that you are set up for it to occur. If you want to get the best results possible from the Seven Stages, it's important that you have all the tools you need and that you understand the actions you should take before you begin and, while you're on the plan, the ones you should follow through with. Let's take a look at these essential elements.

Tools for Success

Get ready to begin the Seven Stages by picking up the following items:

For Eating and Tracking:

- Food scale (preferably electronic)
- Measuring cups and spoons
- Nine-inch plates (Check yours at home first: place a tape measure or ruler across the widest part of the plate)
- A meal tracker, such as our 20/20 LifeStyles app or a physical journal to write your meals in
- A scale and/or a measuring tape

For Exercise (you'll find more information on these items later in the chapter):

- Running shoes
- Heart rate monitor
- Pedometer

Love Diet Action Items—Before You Start the Seven Stages

Research in motivational psychology has revealed that having goals and creating accountability can increase the likelihood of lasting success. And cleaning out your pantry . . . it's obvious why this will be helpful to you! Be sure to complete these three steps before you begin:

- **Establish your goal weight and goal waist measurement:** Setting goals before you start the plan will help ignite your motivation and give you a destination to aim for. We recommend that you aim to lose 1 to 2 percent of your body weight per week. An individual who weighs two hundred pounds, for example, would want to lose two to four pounds per week.
- **Write a contract with yourself:** There is something affirming about putting a commitment to yourself down on paper—it helps the realization that you deserve to be happy, healthy, and loving to yourself truly sink in. Sit down with a pen and a piece of paper and make it official that you're going to change your life starting now. Try writing something specific, for example: *I'm going to eat healthfully every day and exercise five times a week. I'm also going to be kind and loving to myself and others. I am worth the effort and the rewards that will soon be mine: permanent weight loss and long-lasting health and a better outlook for my future.* Be sure to sign and date it, and come back to it whenever you need a reminder of your commitment to yourself.
- **Clean out your pantry:** This is arguably the most important step to complete before you begin the Seven Stages. Even if you think

your favorite snacks will be safe in the back of the cupboard
where you won't see them, they won't.

It's especially important during the first stage of the plan that your pantry be clear of sabotaging foods—chips, crackers, cookies, ice cream, etc. At first, you will be working to restore metabolic balance, and for the first few days you may still be experiencing cravings. To eliminate the temptation, remove sabotaging foods.

When we say your pantry, we really mean anywhere else you might keep food too—this includes your fridge, freezer, office, desk, car, or any other cupboard, nook, or cranny—any place where junk foods, snacks, and other high-calorie treats may be hiding. Enlist the help of your spouse, family members, or friends in this endeavor. You'll be tempted to keep certain foods that belong to someone else in the house—"Those pretzels are for the kids," or "My husband really likes ice cream"—but ultimately your family should want you to be healthy and be willing to do everything they can to support you.

Perhaps now is the time to teach your kids a little more about healthy eating and help them get involved in the process. Depending on how old they are, you can ask them to prep the veggies—even little hands can tear the lettuce for a salad. If anyone in the house resists your request to keep only healthful foods in the house, ask them to eat their snacks or desserts when they're out. This includes asking your loved ones to avoid bringing home treats or desserts from work or social gatherings. Let your significant others know that they can eat those foods at work but to please keep them out of the house. If your family wants ice cream, suggest that they leave the house and go get some. This way, your family can enjoy occasional treats but still support you with a fridge and pantry full of healthful foods.

In each stage chapter, you'll see a list of suggested foods for that particular stage. Let these lists be your grocery guide each week. Let them help you fill your pantry with on-plan foods. (The list of proteins and vegetables on pages 100, 101, and 113 can be used to stock your fridge in every stage of the plan.)

It's important to check your pantry and fridge throughout the program to make sure it stays clear of junk food and snacks. One of the easiest ways to stick to your meal plan is to keep off-plan foods out of the house. The foods in your house should now be a reflection of your healthy lifestyle.

Love Diet Action Items—On the Plan

Developing these habits during the plan and sticking to them will help accelerate and improve your results and will also give you the feedback you need to make adjustments as you go. Let's take a look.

Exercise Regularly

There is a medication on the market for nearly every irritation, condition, or disease that afflicts us. And yet, not one of these medications is as powerful as the act of exercise. Exercise truly is a magic potion: it keeps you young in body and mind, burns calories, and assists in weight loss and weight maintenance. The best part is, it doesn't come with a long list of potential side effects like most medications do. Well, it does have some side effects—but they're all good. Exercise has so many benefits because it:

- Strengthens your heart, lungs, and circulatory system
- Decreases stress
- Lowers inflammation, which can reduce pain and bolster immunity
- Eliminates insulin resistance and improves insulin sensitivity
- Increases productivity, improves sleep, and restores energy
- Boosts mood by turning up production of feel-good neurotransmitters
- Builds and hardens bones
- Improves posture and balance
- Promotes healthy body weight
- Blocks the hardening of arteries

The final point is a big one—every time you exercise, you release nitric oxide (NO) from the cells that line your arteries. These NO molecules then work to relax the blood vessels and help prevent your arteries from stiffening during exercise and for hours after you complete a workout. Healthy and relaxed arteries are one of the keys to lasting health—because hardening here is a primary pathway to coronary heart disease, the number one killer of men and women in this country.

No matter what your starting point, exercise will produce noticeable improvements in how you look and feel. Even if you've been sedentary for years, exercising will quickly begin to work its magic on you, opening your lungs up so that everyday movements and activities feel easier and more enjoyable.

We have divided the exercise recommendations into three categories by fitness level. Read through the categories to see where you would place yourself—be honest and aim to put yourself in the appropriate category, as this will not only help minimize chance of injury but also ensure you're getting the workout you need to help progress your weight loss.

Once you get to the Seven Stages, you'll see the specific workouts for your fitness level within each stage. Stick to the exercise guidelines as best you can and be sure not to overdo it—this can lead to physical exhaustion, which can cause your body to go into starvation mode, stalling weight loss. For all levels, we recommend exercising a minimum of five days per week, but note that bumping this up to six days can accelerate your rate of weight loss.

Take a look at these fitness categories to see where you fit in:

Level 1, Low Fitness or Deconditioned: You likely have a sedentary job and lifestyle. You haven't participated in formal exercise or sports in the last year, and you might find that you get winded walking up two flights of stairs.

Level 2, Moderate Fitness or Fairly Active: You have an active job or lifestyle. You are physically active at least twenty hours per week, or you participate in moderate workouts two to three times per week. You might work a physically demanding job that requires heavy lifting or walking long distances. Your level of fitness allows you to participate in activities that require moderate intensity or output, such as skiing, snowboarding, or basketball.

Level 3, High Fitness or Very Active. You are very physically active. You participate in vigorous activity at least three days per week. This could mean that you run for forty-five minutes, work at least twenty hours per week performing strenuous labor, or play a high-intensity sport two to three days per week. (If you fall in this category, we recommend that you not train for any type of long endurance event while following the Seven Stages—events that demand ninety minutes or more of exercise each day would require a diet different from the one you'll be following in this book.)

In addition to completing the workout for your fitness level during each stage, you will also want to complete the activity listed under "All Levels." Here you will find the recommended number of steps you should walk each day. This number does not count the steps you take during your workout. We want to make sure you are reaching at least five thousand steps per day, and in some stages at least six thousand steps per day. How do you know you're hitting your step goal? You wear a pedometer, which is one of just a few basic tools you'll need to help you stay on track with exercise and movement during the Love Diet (and hopefully beyond). Here are the recommended tools—and one important technique—for fitness success:

Running shoes: You will be spending a lot of time walking or running on this plan, which means you need to make sure you have a good pair of running shoes. A quality pair of shoes will help prevent foot and joint pain and may cost you about $100—this is one area where you don't want to skimp on price. To find the best pair for your foot, gait, weight, and activity level, visit a local sporting goods or running shoe store. If you have known foot issues, we recommend that you try to resolve them before you begin the plan, because exercise is essential to your success. Your primary care physician or a podiatrist can put you on the path to pain-free feet.

Heart rate monitor: Throughout the stages, you will see the instruction to perform an exercise at a level that allows you to reach your optimum heart rate. We use heart rate as a measure of output, with an increase in heart rate suggesting that you're working harder and a decrease in heart rate suggesting that you're slowing down. Reaching your optimum heart rate during exercise is recommended, as this will ensure that you're functioning at a level that is best suited for weight loss. To use your heart rate as an indicator of output, you need two things: to know your goal heart rate and a tool to measure it.

Your goal heart rate while exercising, referred to as optimum heart rate, is determined by a formula based on your age. To figure out your optimum heart rate, take 220 and subtract your age—this is your maximum heart rate. Now, take your maximum heart rate and multiply it by 0.65; this equals the low end or your minimum optimum heart rate. Next, take your maximum heart rate again and multiply it this time by 0.85; this equals the high end or your maximum optimum heart rate (different from your maximum heart rate). Here's an example using a forty-year-old individual:

In this case, you would subtract 40 from 220 and get 180. Then, you would multiply 180 × 0.65, which equals 117—the low end of this person's optimum heart rate. Next, you would multiply 180 × 0.85, which equals 153—the high end of this person's optimum heart rate. These two figures then represent this person's optimum heart rate while exercising; the person wants to make sure to keep their heart rate between 117 and 153.

To measure your heart rate, you will need to pick up a heart rate monitor. There are several good ones on the market today, and they're improving quickly as the technology advances. We like Polar brand watches, which you can find at 2020lifestyles.com, or you can visit a local sporting goods store to try out the options they offer. Some heart rate monitors offer a chest strap, which is more accurate, especially if you plan on running. The most important point is that you find one that's comfortable for you to wear while exercising.

> **Pedometer:** A pedometer is a basic, inexpensive, yet crucial tool that you can use during the Love Diet. You can pick up a wearable pedometer or look for a pedometer feature or app on your smartphone. Tracking your steps and exercise is just as important as tracking your meals—and a pedometer will help you get an accurate picture of how many steps you take each day. Your steps goal during the stages will be a minimum range of five to six thousand steps per day. Remember, these five thousand steps do not include the steps you get while exercising, so remove your pedometer during exercise.

If you're low on steps at the end of a day, find a way to hit your goal—even if it means you have to walk around your house until you reach it (weather and darkness should not be excuses for not getting it done!).

If you exceed the steps goal for the day, know that this will only benefit your weight loss efforts. In fact, many of our participants walk ten thousand or more steps per day to help accelerate their weight loss. Walking is an activity that is difficult to get too much of and will rarely result in overtraining symptoms.

Make sure you have each of these tools before you start the Seven Stages; they'll be vitally important to your success on the program.

Become a Tracker

We cannot stress enough how important tracking will be, not only during the program, but also for at least two years after you reach your goal weight.

It is vital to track the number of calories and protein, fat, and carbohydrates you consume, as well as your portion sizes, including the weight and measurement of foods. Keeping track of this information helps ensure that you are meeting your calorie and protein recommendations and that you're eating precisely what you need to be eating to promote consistent weight loss. Plus, since tracking requires that you to pay close attention to portion size, it also works as an exercise in knowledge building, improving your ability to automatically determine how much of a food you can eat. After a few months of tracking foods religiously, you'll find that recognizing and making the right choices becomes second nature. Nutrition knowledge is a powerful tool, and meal tracking is a great way to learn more about the food you are putting into your body.

You'll also want to track your weight loss weekly. Monitoring these measurements will help give you clear markers of your progress and alert you if your weight loss begins to slow or plateau. If you do notice a change in your progress, look to your meal tracker for clues. What changed this week? Did you add a new food group? Reintroduced foods can cause your metabolism to lag or create digestive issues that impact weight loss. If you think a certain food might be behind your stalled progress, consider removing the food again and be sure to continue to track your results. If your weight loss resumes, keep this food out of your diet for the remainder of the plan.

The more you record in your tracker, the more useful it will be. You can record your steps, sleep, and stress level (to get better at managing stress, see "The Love Diet Guide to Better Sleep and Less Stress" in the Resources section) to help identify how your body and weight loss respond to lifestyle factors other than eating. Let the data guide you toward making the right adjustments to your habits. If too little sleep affects you negatively, perhaps increasing hunger or causing a lag in weight loss, make an extra effort to get more shut-eye; the effort will pay off. Remember, tracking is most effective in changing your behavior if you do it within fifteen minutes of your meal or snack. Waiting until the end of the day or even several days to track meals could result in a less accurate record and impede the program's effectiveness.

There are many ways to track your eating habits. Remember to check out our free 20/20 LifeStyles app or look for other tracking apps online. A journal can work just as well—just make sure you always have it with you!

Drink More Water

It's vitally important that you drink enough water while following the Seven Stages. The changes occurring in your body as you lose weight and balance your metabolism will put additional demands on your hydration. We recommend that you drink at least 64 ounces of water a day; that's eight 8-ounce glasses of water. Almost all of the major systems in your body need water to function, and they need a lot of it if they are to function at their best. Let's look at the specific reasons you'll need more water during the plan:

- **Thirsty muscle doesn't burn calories:** Muscle tissue is the primary calorie burner in your body, and since it's made up of over 70 percent water, it needs plenty of hydration to burn at the maximum rate. When you're not properly hydrated, your muscles' ability to generate energy and burn fat for fuel is severely compromised, and the result is a slowed metabolism. To increase weight loss and metabolism, it's important to keep your muscles hydrated!
- **Increased protein in your diet and fat loss create metabolic waste:** The good news is that this waste is water soluble, which means staying on top of your hydration will help clear these waste products right out of the body.
- **You need healthy blood:** Water is essential to maintaining blood volume, which is vital to muscle efficiency. Without enough blood, your muscles don't get the oxygen and nutrients to function at their best.
- **More fiber equals a greater need for water:** The Seven Stages plan is relatively high in fiber, which will help keep you fuller longer and promote healthy digestion. But more fiber with not enough water is not a good thing, as constipation can result. Get eight glasses in a day to help you stay regular. If you are having constipation problems with the Love Diet, then add a fiber supplement to your meal plan and drink more water.
- **Thirst can often be mistaken for hunger:** We frequently misinterpret thirst for hunger. If at any time during the plan, you feel hungry

and it's not your meal or snack time, drink a big glass of water and then see how you feel.

- **Water increases feelings of fullness:** When you drink water with your meals, not only will you get all the benefits of good hydration but you will also feel fuller sooner.
- **Increased exercise means more sweat:** When you sweat, you lose a great deal of water and key electrolytes that keep your body's function in balance. And since you'll be exercising at least five times a week, there's no doubt that you'll be sweating more. Make sure this water gets replaced by drinking 64 ounces of water a day. This is the equivalent of eight cups of water each day, or approximately six water bottles. If still water is a difficult transition, try sparkling water or noncaloric flavored sparkling water.

So now that you know how much water you should drink and why you should drink it, you're probably wondering *how* to do it. If you've only been drinking a couple glasses of water a day, you'll need to create some new habits to make sure you get more in. Here are six strategies we've found to be successful:

1. **Drink water that tastes good:** It's important to find water that tastes good to you. Depending on where you live, you might be able to drink unfiltered tap water, but in most locations a water filtration system or bottled water will be needed for quality drinking water. Sparkling, nonflavored, or flavored water without added sweeteners can also become your new favorite.
2. **Carry a container with you:** Choose a container that is convenient and attractive. Have it with you all day and train yourself to use it, looking for refill stops. Most coffee shops will refill your water bottle for free, as will bars and restaurants. Even convenience store fountain machines typically have a water lever hidden beneath the soda brands. Simply ask if you can grab some water since you're skipping the soda.
3. **Track water too:** Use your meal tracker to record your water consumption and challenge yourself to hit your goal each day.

4. **Flavor your water:** Use sliced lemon, orange, lime, or cucumber to add a bit of interesting flavor to your water. Fresh herbs like lemon verbena, mint, and stevia leaves can infuse delicate flavors as well. You can also try herbal or decaffeinated teas.
5. **Make it a treat:** When dining out, try carbonated mineral water with a twist of lemon or lime instead of an alcoholic drink. Try different brands, such as San Pellegrino and Perrier, to see if you can find a favorite.
6. **Know that there is no replacement for water:** Caffeine dehydrates you, and soda is loaded with sugar. Sodas and caffeinated drinks such as tea and coffee actually promote water loss in your body; they are not replacements for water.

Remember to Be Mindful

In Chapter 3, we discussed the concept of mindless eating and how destructive it can be to your efforts to lose weight. We also addressed how you can reprogram your habit response to help break mindless eating habits. Here, we'll pick up where that section left off and introduce to you a few other ways to become a more mindful eater, the opposite of a mindless eater.

Mindful eating means that you will slow down your eating to focus on savoring and enjoying your meal. You will focus on the process of eating in order to give your body and your mind a chance to connect with and experience satiety. When you eat too fast, you actually eat beyond fullness simply because you haven't given your body time to process what it's already been given. Here's how to become a more mindful eater:

- **Always make sure water is present:** Water belongs on the table, no matter where you're eating or what you're eating. It should become a constant fixture on your table. Consider getting a nice clear pitcher and filling it with cold water and thinly sliced lemons—talk about an inviting refreshment.

- **Look at your plate of food and appreciate what is in front of you:** Rather than digging in immediately, take a moment to anticipate eating and enjoying your meal.
- **Think of eating as a sensory experience meant to be savored:** It's important to be aware of every bite and how it feels in your mouth, to consider its aromas and appreciate its flavors. As you eat, try to identify some of the spices used in the dish. Most importantly, take your time and enjoy the nourishment you are receiving.
- **Place your fork, spoon, or knife back on the plate between each bite:** Before you pick up your fork, have a sip of water.
- **Be the last one to finish eating:** This might be a new experience for you, but keep in mind that mealtime isn't intended to be a race.
- **Time how long it takes you to eat:** Make a note of how long it takes you to eat a meal, and next time try to go a bit slower. Research shows that slower eaters consume fewer calories.
- **Do not eat in front of the television set, computer, or while working on any other task:** Make eating a food-focused event by eliminating distractions.
- **As always, be sure to meal track:** Tracking will help create a stronger connection with your eating habits.

Incorporating more of these mindful eating techniques will help you automatically remove many of the cues or habits that have been triggering your mindless eating.

Take Your Vitamins

Your body functions at its best when it's fully stocked with all the vitamins, minerals, and antioxidants that are important to your metabolism, digestion, immune health, and more. While the eating plan featured in this book will increase your intake of several important vitamins, amino acids, and phytonutrients (beneficial chemical compounds found in plants)—especially thanks to the steady intake of lean proteins and vegetables after the first stage—supplementing your diet can help ensure that you have everything you need for optimum health and results.

We recommend that you take at least a multivitamin, fish oil, and vitamin D_3. Going beyond that can be helpful but not entirely essential unless you have a known clinical deficiency. If you are interested in supplementing further, check out "Extended Supplement Section" on page 291. You can find our line of supplements in the 20/20 LifeStyles store online, or you can pick up any of these at a local supplement store—just be sure to select a reputable brand to ensure you're getting what you pay for.

Multivitamin: A good-quality multivitamin is recommended while you're following the Love Diet and beyond—it can help keep you healthier by filling in nutritional gaps in your diet. Look for one that contains vitamins C, D_3, E, and the B vitamins of folic acid, B_6, and B_{12}.

Fish oil: We refer to fish oil as the fountain of youth because it can slow the aging process and prevent many disorders. It helps prevent heart disease, type 2 diabetes, and high blood pressure. It also has a powerful anti-inflammatory effect that can benefit your brain and joints.

The protective powers of fish oil were noted by a Danish scientist who observed that the Greenland Eskimos had an exceptionally low incidence of heart disease and arthritis despite eating a very high-fat diet consisting largely of whale blubber.

Researchers have found that fish is very high in two essential omega-3 fatty acids called EPA and DHA. They are called essential fatty acids because our bodies cannot make them, yet they're essential in preventing aging of our cells and hardening of our arteries. In order to get them, we have to incorporate omega-3 fatty acids and other essential fatty acids into our diet—either in foods that contain them or supplements that do.

Look for a fish oil blend that is fresh, purified (free of heavy metals), and will provide you with around 600 milligrams of EPA and 400 milligrams of DHA.

Vitamin D_3: We have found that most of our 20/20 LifeStyles participants are low in this important vitamin. Our bodies produce vitamin D_3 from sunlight, but the production can be diminished by the use of sunscreen, which is important to reduce the risk of skin cancer. If you live in a sunny climate and are outdoors a great deal of the time, you probably don't need to take additional vitamin D_3, but even then it's worth having your doctor check your levels.

Vitamin D_3 may help improve insulin sensitivity, can benefit your immune system, and will assist in the absorption of calcium and phosphorous, both of which are important to bone health. We recommend 400 IU daily for adults and 600 IU daily for seniors.

And One Last Tool for Success: The Right Attitude

It's often our thoughts that sabotage our best dieting efforts, so getting into the right mental space before you begin is just as important as picking up all the tools you'll need for the plan.

Throughout the book, you've learned how important your mind is to creating the life you want—you know that a Slimming Mindset will help free you from any feelings of guilt and shame about your eating and your weight, and that banishing negative self-talk and practicing more positive mantras will increase your feelings of self-love and self-respect.

Similarly, it's important to surrender two thoughts that we often hear people express as they're on the brink of beginning the Love Diet. The first is, *If I can't stick to the plan perfectly, then I might as well give up,* and the second is, *I can't believe I'm about to start yet another diet.* Let's quickly break down why these have got to go:

Perfection isn't possible: Don't set yourself up for failure from the beginning by having overly rigid and strict expectations. The Love Diet shouldn't be approached with an all-or-nothing diet mentality but rather with one that allows you to overcome any lapses and develop the skill of getting yourself back on track. This is especially important if you're an emotional eater because you're more likely to let just one slipup spiral into several. Take it one meal at a time, and if you eat off plan, don't dwell on it—just make a promise to do better at your next meal. Leave the past in the past and focus on what you can do in the present moment that's best for your health.

Not just another diet—your last diet: You may be thinking that the last thing you want to do is start another diet. You might have even started convincing yourself that your current weight isn't so bad and that you've gotten used to being heavier and dealing with the physical challenges and discomforts associated with your weight. If you find thoughts such as these starting to sneak into your head, pause to see if they pass the truth test. Are you truly happy with your life as you're currently living it? Are you willing to continue to accept the health risks and other burdens that come with excess weight? If you answer honestly, we think you'll find that change and a better life are your destiny—so don't deny yourself this chance to seize them. And remember that the diet you're following in this book has been the last diet for thousands of successful individuals. Now it's your turn to start the last diet you'll ever need. Let's get started.

PART III

The Seven Stages and Beyond

You're officially ready to begin the Seven Stages. Congratulations! In the following chapters, we will guide you through the eating plan, which will help transform your body one stage at a time. We will use the first stage to simplify your diet to include only a select group of metabolically balancing foods. During this stage, you will experience a profound reset of your metabolic system, which controls your hunger, cravings, and metabolism. If you have struggled with weight loss for some time, this metabolic reboot will be critical to your success because it will help correct any possible underlying metabolic imbalances.

During the subsequent stages, you will gradually add back in other types of foods such as vegetables, certain types of dairy, fruit, and more. As you do, it's important to pay attention to how your body responds to each reintroduced food. If you notice problems such as bloating, weight gain, or digestive discomfort after you add a specific food back into your diet, you will want to consider removing that food again temporarily (or for good, like Kim did with grains; see page 68). This will ultimately allow you to create a personalized diet that works best for your body. Most people go their entire lives without identifying their problem foods, but that doesn't mean you have to; the Seven Stages will put you in the driver's seat of your diet destiny.

Each of the Seven Stages will focus on one type of food, but that's not all you'll eat—this isn't the cabbage soup diet! Your meals will be rounded out with strategically selected foods that will help promote weight loss and keep you satiated. Be sure to visit the Love Diet Meal

Plans chapter as you progress through the program. You will find three days' worth of meals for each stage there.

A Quick Note Before You Begin

If you haven't read through the previous chapters, we strongly encourage you to go back and do so. It's there that you will learn how vitally important self-love and a Slimming Mindset are to your weight loss journey—these truly are critical components of lasting weight loss success; they will provide you with the emotional foundation you need to commit to and follow through with the dietary changes you are about to make.

You'll also find some of our success stories there, which will help you see the possibilities for life on the other side of the Seven Stages. What incredible adventures and opportunities are waiting for you? When you follow the Seven Stages and develop a renewed sense of self-love, you give yourself the chance to take ten years off your life, just like Donna did; she said she has never felt younger or looked better than after the plan. You could also go from being 310 pounds to climbing a fourteen-thousand-foot mountain, which is what Kurt was able to do after he followed the Seven Stages. Or, like Evan, you might go from being a lifelong yo-yo dieter to someone who starts with small changes and then works his way up to a hundred-pound weight loss. You might also discover how specific foods affect how you feel, not unlike Kim, in order to make the necessary changes to improve your health and life. The possibilities for creating your new life story are endless. Welcome to a new era of loving yourself and gifting yourself (finally) with the health you deserve! Now, let's get started with the stages.

CHAPTER 6

Stage 1: Detox

Stage 1 marks the beginning of your journey back to health. As you embark on this journey, remember why you are here: to put the self-love that's blossoming inside of you to work! Use this powerful force of care and compassion to motivate you to start and stick with the eating plan you'll discover on the following pages. Every effort you make to fill your body with healthful foods is a reflection of love, not limitation. Recognize that instead of holding back the pleasure of processed foods, you're rewarding yourself with lifelong health, the greatest gift of all.

This first one-week stage will help reset your body's metabolic system so that you are no longer battling cravings and hunger. Years of eating a diet high in simple and refined carbohydrates has likely left you with dysfunctional appetite hormones, which set you up to overeat, and chronically high insulin levels, which trigger your body to perpetually store fat and contribute to fatigue and irritability. Because you will not lose weight under these metabolic conditions, Stage 1 will work to correct imbalances, unlocking weight loss and producing other noticeable benefits such as increased energy and improved moods.

The primary goal during this stage is to regain control of your blood sugar levels. You want your blood sugar to work like a smooth flight on an airplane—it should go up and come down gradually, not quickly or chaotically. Turbulence here is the catalyst of nearly all metabolic dysfunction that leads to weight gain.

Stage 1 is centered on lean and very lean protein, healthy fats, and berries. It's important to note that this means you will be removing all grains and starches from your diet. This includes all breads, pastas, crackers, cookies, candies, chips, and baked goods. Although this may seem restrictive, eating berries along with the right type of proteins and fats will meet your body's nutritional and satiety needs for the first week. These dietary staples will help your body detoxify, jump-starting your weight loss. And you'll be pleasantly surprised at how after a few days, you won't even feel tempted by sweets, fatty meats, or other processed foods. Let's take a closer look at the nutritional stars of this stage.

Berries

Berries will be your main carbohydrate source for the first few stages of the meal plan. Berries are the ultimate superfood. They provide excellent energy to the body and fuel to the brain; they're rich in detoxifying antioxidants, and they contain natural anti-inflammatory properties. Further, because they're lower in carbohydrates than other fruits, they don't contribute to blood sugar imbalances or elevated blood insulin levels. For all these reasons, we'd like you to think of berries as their own food group and even consider them your safe carbohydrate.

Throughout the stages, you will be encouraged to eat one-cup servings of berries, sometimes as often as four to five times a day. The allotted servings of berries in the meal plan will provide you with the carbohydrates you need for energy throughout the day without triggering intense cravings or hunger.

In this stage, eat plenty of fresh or frozen blueberries, blackberries, raspberries, and strawberries, but omit cranberries due to their high sugar content. If you choose frozen berries, be sure to select berries that are unsweetened or without any added syrup or sugar.

Lean and Very Lean Proteins

You may remember from Chapter 4 that proteins will be an important part of your diet during the Seven Stages. Foods with protein will keep you fuller longer and, in the process, help your body repair and reset itself during this critical first stage. We've separated proteins into two categories: lean and very lean. The difference between the two is the fat content of very lean is lower than lean. Very lean proteins actually don't have enough fat to meet your body's needs, so when you eat these proteins, you will need to add a serving of healthy fat. The key is to make sure you're adding the right kind of fat and in the right amount—we'll provide you with specifics in the next section starting on page 101. Lean proteins have adequate fat content, so there is no need for you to add additional fat when enjoying these foods. Sorry, bacon lovers, if your favorite protein is not on the list, avoid it during the early stages of our plan.

One type of protein that you should minimize while following the Seven Stages is processed meats. Due to their high sodium content, you should eat these sparingly, and if you have high blood pressure, you should avoid them completely. Processed meats include: deli meats, such as packaged sliced turkey or ham and all sliced meats from the deli case; precooked packaged meats, such as refrigerated chicken or steak strips; and most frozen proteins, such as breakfast sausage, turkey or salmon burgers, precooked meatballs, and so on.

If you do use processed meat or fish to satisfy your protein requirement for a meal, be sure to select varieties that have less than 500 milligrams of sodium per serving and eat them with only one meal per day. Limiting processed meats to one meal per day will help you keep your sodium in your target range of 1,500 to 2,300 milligrams per day. Be wary of serving sizes here—if one serving is only 2 ounces of protein and 450 milligrams of sodium, and you need 4 ounces for your meal, you would end up consuming 900 milligrams of sodium. In this example, this particular processed meat would not fit into your meal plan.

To avoid relying on processed meats as your primary source of protein, consider batch cooking better-quality, approved proteins. One or two nights a week, grill or bake enough chicken breasts or lean steaks to last you through the week. This will save you time with meal prep and planning and will make sure you're not stuck relying on processed meats for protein.

Your protein serving sizes for the first three stages will be as listed in the chart on the following page. The ounce measurements refer to cooked weight.

STAGES 1–3 PROTEIN SERVING SIZES

Women

- 4 ounces for breakfast
- 4 ounces for lunch
- 6 ounces for dinner

Men

- 4 ounces for breakfast
- 6 ounces for lunch
- 8 ounces for dinner

During the Seven Stages, you will have a big selection of proteins with which to make your meals. This list will be consistent throughout the program:

Very Lean Proteins: Chicken breast (skinless); turkey breast (skinless); low-sodium deli chicken or turkey; canned tuna (limit to two servings per week); fresh or frozen tilapia, cod, or halibut; fresh or frozen shrimp; ground beef (4–5%); venison; bison; and liquid egg whites, egg beaters, or egg substitutes

Lean Proteins: Salmon, pork tenderloin, lean beef (sirloin steak; flank steak; tenderloin; and rib, chuck, or rump roast), low-sodium deli ham, ground beef (7–10%), and dark-meat poultry without skin

If you do not eat meat or fish, there are vegetarian protein options that you can eat during the Seven Stages. It is, however, important to follow our selection guidelines for vegetarian sources of protein. Most importantly, you have to check the label to make sure you're getting adequate protein. Most vegetarian options will only have the protein listed in grams instead of ounces, but that's okay—a quick calculation will tell us how many grams you need to meet the ounce requirement. There are 7 grams of protein in each ounce, which means if you need

4 ounces of protein, you'll need to make sure you're getting 28 grams ($7 \times 4 = 28$) and if you need 6 ounces, you'll need to get 42 grams of protein ($7 \times 6 = 42$).

Here are your vegetarian protein options:

Vegetarian Very Lean Proteins: High-protein tofu from brands such as Azumaya Lite and Sol Cuisine, and foods made from TVP (texturized vegetable protein)

Vegetarian Lean Protein Options: Soy products such as burgers or patties;* mock deli meats, meatballs, and hot dogs made by brands like Boca, MorningStar Farms, and Beyond Meat; high-protein tofu from Wildwood or Nutrela; and tempeh

Healthy Fats

Unsaturated dietary fats, such as plant oils, avocados, and nuts, do more than promote a healthy heart and increase levels of good cholesterol (not to mention, taste great)—they also provide protective nutrients important for the body's absorption of key antioxidants and vitamins, and they may even help increase satiety. Medical research also suggests healthful dietary fat may decrease risk factors associated with type 2 diabetes.

You will be adding one healthy fat serving to your very lean proteins at breakfast, lunch, and dinner. Each fat serving should be 45 calories and provide 5 grams of fat.

Here are several healthy fat options (add to very lean protein only):

- 1 teaspoon plant-based oil such as canola, peanut, or extra-virgin olive oil
- 2 teaspoons natural peanut, almond, or nut butter (no added sugar or oil on the ingredients label)

* Avoid garden burger style, as they may contain grains

- 1 tablespoon low-fat mayonnaise
- 1 tablespoon seeds (sesame, sunflower, pumpkin)
- 2 tablespoons low-fat salad dressing
- ⅛ avocado
- 6 almonds
- 10 peanuts
- 10 black olives

How to Enhance Your Meals

You can use a wide variety of herbs, spices, and salt-free spice blends freely during the Seven Stages. We encourage you to add these to your meals when you feel you need to wake up your palate a bit.

> **Calorie-Free Flavor Boosters***: Lemon or lime juice or zest, garlic, ginger, green onions, parsley, red pepper flakes, basil, oregano, mustard, cumin, paprika, and all varieties of vinegars.

Beverages

Of course, it's also nice to enjoy a meal with a refreshing beverage. Since you'll be removing all calorie-containing beverages (except for protein shakes; see sidebar) during the Seven Stages—this means no alcohol or sugar-sweetened beverages such as juice or soda—we suggest healthier alternatives that won't sabotage your weight loss efforts. It's important to keep calorie-containing beverages out of your diet because they don't contribute to satiety, meaning they don't fill you up despite the fact that they provide a high number of calories.

* If you use any spice blends, eliminate those that contain any form of sugar or salt as an ingredient.

DRINKING PROTEIN SHAKES ON THE PLAN

Throughout the Seven Stages, you'll notice "20/20 High Protein Dry Powder Breakfast Shake" and "20/20 High Protein Ready to Drink Breakfast Shake" listed as breakfast and snack options. These shakes are optional to enjoy during the eating plan and can be purchased at 2020lifestyles.com. Because these have been designed specifically to help individuals following our plan, with the ideal number of calories and the perfect balance of protein and carbs, we can't recommend an alternative shake that can be purchased in stores. However, the whole-foods based options listed in the nutrition specifics section will work just as well in helping restore and maintain metabolic balance.

To enjoy a 20/20 High Protein Dry Powder Breakfast Shake, blend the following ingredients until smooth, and drink cold:

1 cup ice

1 cup berries, fresh or frozen

1 cup water

1 packet 20/20 LifeStyles Protein Powder

For the 20/20 High Protein Ready to Drink Breakfast Shake, serve chilled with 1 cup of berries on the side. When you enjoy either of these options as your breakfast, you will also add 1 tablespoon of nut butter.

Beverage Options: Mineral water, Talking Rain with fruit essence (without any sweetener), herbal tea, decaf coffee, and green or white tea. Caffeinated beverages can be consumed, but with limits: coffee intake should not exceed 8 ounces of black drip coffee or two shots of espresso per day, and regular tea should be limited to 16 ounces per day.

The one beverage that is included on the plan and that you should drink as often as possible is water. Water intake is crucial for regulating body temperature and nutrient transport, and for helping rebalance the good bacteria in your intestinal tract. It also can help you feel fuller, which will work in your favor, especially during this first stage as you adjust to a new way of eating. Aim to drink 64 ounces of water per day. The best way to start drinking more water is to make sure you always have some with you. Pick up a reusable container and take advantage of drinking fountains and water coolers, and when you're on the go, don't be afraid to ask at coffee shops, restaurants, bars, and convenience stores if there's somewhere you can fill your water bottle. Add a slice of lemon or lime, even sliced cucumber, or fresh herbs like lemon verbena, mint, and stevia. All of these fresh additions will give your water a little burst of flavor.

Putting It All Together

Since your goal during the Seven Stages is to produce steady weight loss, you will need to pay attention to calories. Throughout the program, we recommend that women eat between 1,100 and 1,400 calories each day, while men should eat between 1,300 and 1,700 calories each day. Do not eat less than the minimum recommended number of calories! This will only program your body to feel as though it's starving—when your body senses starvation, it will do everything it can to hold on to excess weight.

It's also important to make sure you eat at regular intervals. Avoid skipping meals or snacks. When you miss meals or snacks, you're more likely to lose control of your hunger and cravings and to make poor choices. Aim to eat a meal or snack every three to four hours.

What to Expect

If you're feeling a little nervous or anxious about starting Stage 1, you're not alone—many of our participants expressed similar feelings before beginning. (Revisiting positive self-talk techniques can help here; see page 47.) The good news is that most of them come back the second week saying that it was much easier than expected. That's because the meal plan is easy to follow: it offers you clear structure and guidelines on what to eat in order to reset your metabolic functions and jump-start your weight loss.

Remember to make sure you're eating enough calories and to always get the recommended amount of protein each day. This is essential to your success. Without enough protein, you'll feel hungry and you won't be providing your body with the materials it needs to repair and reset your system. Don't be afraid of experimenting a little in the kitchen; add some of your favorite herbs and spices, or try new ones listed in Chapter 14.

The first three days of the plan may be tough, but there is no doubt that you can do it. You might experience mild headaches, fatigue, and some hunger during the first three days as your body learns to adjust to the new diet. This is natural and to be expected, as these can be side effects of your body detoxing. If you experience any of these sensations, check on your meal frequency and make certain you are getting the right amount of berries—these are your main source of carbohydrates in the first week. They will help boost your energy and keep hunger at bay.

After just a few days, you'll feel much better and won't experience any abnormal levels of hunger. And after seven days, you'll start to feel like a new person. This is no exaggeration—we have seen incredible changes take place in just one week. People who've followed the meal plan and exercised five to six times during Stage 1 have reported:

- More energy and mental clarity than they've felt in a long time
- A disappearance of the fatigue and funk they could never seem to shake
- A decline in elevated blood pressure
- Balanced blood sugar levels
- Between five and eight pounds of weight lost (dependent upon starting weight) and a slimmer waist

If you embrace the meal plan completely and are consistent with exercise, you will experience similarly impressive results in just seven days. It's your turn! Congratulations on taking your first step to a happier and healthier you.

FREQUENTLY ASKED QUESTION: CAN I DINE OUT THIS WEEK?

The first seven days of the Love Diet are critically important to balancing your blood sugar and resetting your metabolic systems. They are so important that we recommend not dining out at this stage—there are too many temptations, and you lose control over what's in and on your food. Still, we know that for some of you, it may not be possible to avoid restaurants completely. If dining out is necessary, here are some tips on how to dine out and still stay on plan:

Make sure you've eaten enough that day: Going out to eat when you're very hungry is a very bad idea—you can't rely on extreme hunger to make smart eating choices for you. If you know you're eating out later in the day, be sure to eat all of your Stage 1 meals and snacks on time.

Know before you go: Just because you're dining out at a restaurant doesn't mean your meals will change—you will still be eating a lean or very lean protein with a healthy serving of fat and one serving of berries. To keep it simple, order a 4- to 6-ounce filet mignon, sirloin, flatiron, or flank steak or a 4- to 6-ounce piece of salmon or other type of fish. Ask for it to be prepared without butter, oil, or sauces. Ordering a lean protein (versus a very lean protein) will provide you with both the protein and fat you need for the meal. Keep in mind that a serving of meat or fish is about the size of a deck of cards or the palm of your hand. If the serving is too large, simply cut it down to size as soon as it's served to you and push the excess to the side of the plate. Then, save the extra portion for tomorrow's lunch.

Stage 1 Nutrition Summary

The plan for this week is designed to be simple and easy to follow. When in doubt, return to this list of the seven dietary changes you will be making for the seven days of Stage 1. We recommend that you flag or note this page so that you always know where it is when you need it:

- Make sure to eat at least 1,100 daily calories for women and 1,300 daily calories for men.

"Save my sides for someone else": When the waiter asks you about potatoes or other tempting side dishes, remember that you've decided to respect and love your body. Your food choices are a reflection of that respect and love. Simply say, "No sides for me, please," or offer them to someone else at the table.

No wine, no beer, no exceptions: If you're asked about a drink, have sparkling water with a twist of lemon or lime. In Stage 1, your body is detoxifying and increasing your metabolism's ability to burn more calories; alcohol will stop that process and stall weight loss. One way to make it easier to not drink is to volunteer to be the designated driver.

Be unabashed about your self-love: If you feel pressure to have a drink or to eat something off plan, remain assertive but gracious in your refusal. "No, thank you" should suffice, even if you have to repeat it a couple of times. If someone makes a comment about you being on another diet, simply point out that you've made a commitment to making better choices every day and you'd appreciate everyone respecting your commitment. Remember, you are showing yourself love by eating only those foods that will bring your body back to health.

Let go of your fear of missing out: Here's an interesting test: try to remember what you ate the last time you dined out. You'll probably have difficulty remembering. That's because you're more likely to remember the conversations or the connections you made with people, not with the food on your plate. During the Love Diet, try to focus more on these connections, whether you're at a restaurant, your office, or at home. What might seem like a distraction at first could end up helping you form closer relationships, all while deepening your commitment to yourself.

- Eat three meals and one snack for women, two snacks for men, as directed. Don't deviate from the plan!
- Eliminate all sodas, diet sodas, and alcohol from your diet.
- Limit yourself to one cup of regular coffee per day (we do not recommend using artificial sweeteners, but if you need to use one, you may use up to one serving of stevia per day).
- Consume 64 ounces of water daily.

STAGE 1 NUTRITION SPECIFICS

Since Stage 1 includes just protein, healthy fats, and berries, it should be relatively easy to remember what you should be eating. In this section, we've laid it out in more detail so you can see precisely what you should be eating each meal and the approximate calories and fat grams you'll want to aim for.

Women: 1,100–1,400 calories per day
Men: 1,300–1,700 calories per day

BREAKFAST:	CALORIES	FAT (G)
4 ounces very lean protein	140	0–4
2 servings healthy fat (page 101)	90	10
1 cup berries	80	0
OR: 20/20 High Protein Dry Powder Breakfast Shake made with 1 cup berries and 1 tablespoon nut butter	360	10
OR: 20/20 High Protein Ready to Drink Breakfast Shake served with 1 cup berries and 1 tablespoon nut butter	309	14

LUNCH:	CALORIES	FAT (G)
WOMEN: 4 ounces very lean/lean protein	140–220	0–12
MEN: 6 ounces very lean/lean protein	210–330	0–18

- Consistently track your meals and snacks on your 20/20 LifeStyles app or another meal tracker.
- Take a daily gender-specific vitamin (see page 92 for supplement recommendations).

Stage 1 Exercise Plan: Start Moving!

Hopefully, you've picked up a good-quality pair of running shoes and you're ready to begin exercising! The goal for your exercise in this stage is simply to get moving. Stick with this simple exercise routine to avoid doing too much, too soon.

The exercise guidelines in the Love Diet are created specifically to help you meet your goals—if you exercise more or less than the suggested durations, your results may suffer. Too little exercise won't help your metabolic functions improve, while too much exercise will cause your body to go into starvation mode and slow your weight loss. Too

	CALORIES	FAT (G)
1 serving healthy fat (for very lean protein only)	45	5
1 cup berries	80	0

DINNER:	**CALORIES**	**FAT (G)**
WOMEN: 6 ounces very lean/lean protein	140–220	0–12
MEN: 8 ounces very lean/lean protein	210–330	0–18
1 serving healthy fat (for very lean protein only)	45	5
1 cup berries	80	0

SNACK

WOMEN: 1 per day between lunch and dinner
MEN: 2 per day; 1 between breakfast and lunch, and 1 between lunch and dinner

Select one of these options per snack:	**CALORIES**	**FAT (G)**
2 ounces very lean protein + 1 cup berries	130	0–2
20/20 High Protein Dry Powder Breakfast Shake made with 1 cup berries (no nut butter)	260	0
20/20 High Protein Ready to Drink Breakfast Shake served with 1 cup berries (no nut butter)	220	6

much exercise can also lead to injury, which will be sure to have an impact on your progress. Remember, we want this lifestyle to last. Following our guidelines that have been created by professionals in exercise science will help prepare your body for the physical challenges to come.

For Stage 1, exercise will be as follows:

Level 1, Low Fitness: Moderate-speed walking, 20 minutes, at least 5 days per week. Moderate means breathing hard but having enough breath to speak in full sentences.

Level 2, Moderate Fitness: High-speed walking 30 minutes, at least 5 days per week. Aim to reach the mid-range of your optimum heart rate.

Level 3, High Fitness: Running 30 minutes, at least 5 days per week. Aim to get your heart rate within your optimum range. If you are already doing more than this, continue to do it.

All Levels: Wear a pedometer each day (remove when exercising), aiming to reach at least 5,000 steps per day, excluding exercise.

Stage 1 Lifestyle Plan: A New Priority: You

While following the Seven Stages requires you to make significant changes to your health habits, you might notice that the biggest shift of all is to your priorities. Instead of putting yourself last on the list, you are now putting yourself first (or you've at least moved up a few positions!). While this might feel uncomfortable at first—especially if you are codependent or used to putting everyone else's needs in front of your own—making yourself a priority will be essential to your success.

You might meet some resistance to this adjustment initially; your kids, significant other, and even some of your friends might tug at your attention and try to pull you away from what you need to do to eat well and exercise regularly. This is when you need to remind them (and yourself) that your commitment will result in a reward for everyone: a happier, healthier, and more energetic version of you. A *you* whose future is filled with exciting possibilities instead of medical scares and health problems.

CHAPTER 7

Stage 2: Veggie Boost

Congratulations—the most difficult part of the Love Diet is now behind you! The first week demanded new lifestyle adjustments, and these likely came with some discomfort—it's never easy to leave your comfort zone (or comfort foods) behind. But you succeeded, and you should be proud of the love, respect, and care you've directed your own way over the past week. You've accomplished so much already, and you're only just getting started.

As you continue to honor your commitment to yourself during this stage, you might encounter some pushback from family, friends, or coworkers, and that's okay—they're still getting used to you setting boundaries and putting yourself first. To help them (and you) adjust, continue to be open and communicative about your process, and whenever possible, invite them to join you for a healthful meal or a walk. This will help break down any feelings of isolation and perhaps even earn you some companions on this journey—or at the very least, some cheerleaders.

Now, let's get to building upon the foundation you've set with Stage 1 and continue making progress with your weight loss and health improvements.

Your North Star Stage

The Stage 2 nutritional guidelines will provide you with meals that are nutritionally complete, healthful, and satisfying. You should consider

WAS STAGE 1 EVERYTHING YOU DESERVE?

Before you move fully into Stage 2, it's important to pause and take an honest look back at your first seven days on the plan. If you didn't see the results you wanted, there's a reason. Did you track your meals and snacks completely? Were you able to exercise five to six times during the first stage? Did you get your five thousand steps in every day? Did you eat every three to four hours as a way to prevent excessive hunger caused by blood sugar imbalance? Did you get enough sleep each night?

If your first week was a disappointment or if life got in the way, we suggest repeating Stage 1. If you spent too much time off plan, then you may not have undergone a metabolic reset, which is critical to your success moving forward. There's no shame in starting over. You deserve nothing but the best from your efforts.

this stage your North Star of the Seven Stages. This means that if at any point within the following stages you feel yourself slipping too far from the plan and your body begins to feel out of balance or your weight starts creeping back up, you can return to Stage 2 to get yourself back on track. It's simple: add nonstarchy vegetables to your proteins, healthy fats, and berries, and soon you will find everything comes back into focus and your progress resumes.

Nonstarchy Vegetables

Stage 2 will bring a burst of flavor, color, and texture with the introduction of nonstarchy vegetables such as leafy greens, asparagus, zucchini, and broccoli. You probably never thought you'd be so excited to be adding vegetables to your plate! Vegetables will not only liven up your diet with some variety, but they'll also provide you with plenty of vitamins, minerals, and fiber. With only 15 to 30 calories per serving, nonstarchy vegetables will increase the volume of your meals while having little impact on your daily caloric intake.

The only significant change in this stage is the addition of nonstarchy vegetables. You will continue eating protein, healthy fats, and berries, just as you did in Stage 1. The great thing about this is you're

THE PROBLEM WITH STARCH

It's best to think of *starch* and *sugar* as synonymous because your body's metabolism reacts to them in a similar way; both will lead to cravings for more carbohydrates, and for many of us, they can contribute to elevated blood sugar levels. Even the starch found in starchy vegetables can break down rapidly into sugar once in the body, which is why you'll want to avoid eating veggies high in starch during the first six stages of the plan.

likely getting really good at making sure you eat these three foods with every meal—so just keep going! To this healthy trio, both men and women will add at least three servings of nonstarchy vegetables. And that's three servings with lunch *and* dinner, for a total of six servings a day. Starchy vegetables like corn, peas, potatoes, sweet potatoes, and winter squash will remain out of your diet for now (they'll be added back in during Stage 7). If six servings per day seems like too much food, you can start with two servings and work your way up. If six servings seems like too little food—and you find that you are still hungry at meals—you can eat as many servings as you'd like of nonstarchy vegetables.

You will have a wide variety of vegetables to add to your meals during this stage:*

Leafy Greens (1 serving = 1½ cups): Lettuce: romaine, red or green leaf, Bibb; escarole, arugula, endive, watercress, radicchio, and spinach

Green Vegetables (1 serving = ½ cup cooked): Artichoke, asparagus, broccoli†, Brussels sprouts†, bok choy, collard greens†, mustard greens†, green beans, kale, and zucchini

Others (1 serving = ½ cup cooked / 1 cup raw): bean sprouts, beets, bell peppers, cabbage, carrots†, cauliflower†, celery, cucumber, eggplant,

* The † indicates that these vegetables are high in fiber. Try to include at least one serving of a high-fiber vegetable each day.

jicama, leeks, mushrooms, onions, radishes, tomatoes (technically a fruit), spaghetti squash, yellow squash, and water chestnuts

New Healthy Fats: Salad Dressing, Sauces, and Marinades

Salad dressings, sauces, and marinades are not required items in Stage 2, but if you would like to include them, you can as long as you count your selection as your fat serving for the meal (exception to this rule noted below).

Pay attention to detail when you add any of these liquids to your meals—they can be sneaky sources of excess calories, so getting used to checking nutrition labels is essential. Check the label and make sure all dressings, sauces, or marinades meet these per-serving guidelines before you use them:

Less than 6 grams of sugar

Less than 6 grams of fat

Less than 550 milligrams of sodium

It's also important to make sure you're only getting one serving per meal; most sauces, marinades, and dressings use a serving size of one tablespoon, but always double-check the label to make sure.

The most important rule with salad dressing is to always get your salads with dressing on the side. Then, use the fork trick to make sure you get added flavor without excessive calories. To use the fork trick, simply dip your fork in the salad dressing before you pick up a bite of salad. Do not build a salad bite and then dip in the dressing—it should be alphabetical: dressing first and then salad.

If you decide to use a fat-free dressing, or a fat-free tomato or marinara sauce, you can still include a separate healthy fat serving with your meal. Limit any fat-free additions to just one serving per meal and make sure your selection meets the sugar and salt guidelines for dressings and sauces.

You can make homemade dressings, sauces, and marinades (see Chapter 14), or you can find options at the store like the following:

MARINADES

A.1.: Marinade

Lawry's: Santa Fe Chili, Caribbean Jerk, Lemon Pepper, Steak & Chop, Baja Chipotle, Herb and Garlic

Masa's: Curry Coconut Sauce, Thai Peanut Sauce

SOY SAUCE*

Bragg Liquid Aminos (found near the soy sauces in the grocery store)

Kroger: Lite Soy Sauce

Yamasa: Less Salt Soy Sauce

MAYONNAISE

Hellmann's: Light Mayonnaise

Kraft: Fat Free or Light Mayonnaise

TOMATO SAUCE

Emeril's: Kicked Up Tomato

Muir Glen: All varieties

SALAD DRESSINGS**

Annie's Naturals: Lite Raspberry Vinaigrette, Tuscany Italian, Lite Gingerly Vinaigrette, Lite Honey Mustard Vinaigrette

Trader Joe's: Champagne Pear Vinaigrette, Asian Style Spicy Peanut Vinaigrette

Kraft: Lite Zesty Italian, Lite Raspberry Vinaigrette, Fat Free Honey Dijon, Fat Free Zesty Italian, Zesty Italian, Sun Dried Tomato Vinaigrette

Newman's Own: Light Italian, Light Balsamic Vinaigrette, Light Lime Vinaigrette, Light Raspberry & Walnut

---

* If you buy soy sauce not found on this list, be sure it has less than 550 mg of sodium per serving.

** If you buy a salad dressing not found on this list, be sure it does not contain yogurt or cheese. These items will be added back in Stage 3.

How to Make Vegetables the Best Part of Your Meals

If you're not a fan of vegetables, we hope to turn you into one during the Seven Stages. Vegetables get a bad rap, but most often it's not about the vegetables but actually about other factors that get overlooked. Before you decide you don't like a certain vegetable, ask yourself three questions:

1. Is it in season?
2. It is seasoned?
3. Was it cooked properly to bring out its full flavor?

A "no" in any of these cases might turn you away from a vegetable unnecessarily and prevent you from getting more vitamins, minerals, phytochemicals, and antioxidants into your diet. Let's look at how considering these three questions can improve a vegetable's likeability.

Is It in Season?

Selecting your vegetables according to the season will allow you to take advantage of fruits and vegetables at their peak freshness and quality; this can make all the difference in flavor and even cut down on the need for seasonings or other toppings. If a vegetable isn't in season, you might want to look to the frozen section—frozen vegetables are usually picked during the peak season and then frozen. Here is a quick reference guide for enjoying vegetables (and the fruits, tomato and avocado)* when they're at their best:

Spring: Asparagus, onions, artichokes, strawberries, cantaloupe, papaya, and pineapple

Summer: Tomatoes, squash, bell peppers, eggplant, leafy greens, melons, berries, peaches, apricots, cherries, and grapes

* The † indicates starchy vegetables, which will be eliminated until Stage 7.

Fall: Broccoli, carrots, cauliflower, spinach, pumpkin, sweet potatoes†, beets, kale, apples, bananas, oranges, pears, kiwi, grapefruit, and tangerines

Winter: Snow peas†, winter squash (acorn, butternut, pumpkin)†, radishes, Brussels sprouts, and avocado

Is It Seasoned?

We recommend seasoning vegetables with a pinch of kosher salt and freshly ground black pepper (if you have high blood pressure, omit the salt); a pinch is less than one-tenth of a teaspoon. Add these two seasonings during the cooking process, not at the end, so they can really blend in and boost flavors. You can also use fresh herbs like thyme, basil, dill, mint, parsley, cilantro, oregano, and tarragon to add salt-free flavor. A squeeze or several of fresh lime or lemon juice can brighten a dish of vegetables, and even a splash of vinegar, such as balsamic, sherry, or any wine vinegar, can add a bit of tang without any additional sodium or calories.

Was It Cooked Properly?

How a vegetable is cooked can make all the difference in whether you like it or not—boiled carrots might seem flavorless and mushy to you, but roasted carrots pack a surprisingly sweet and delicious punch. Pairing the right cooking technique with the right type of vegetable will result in satisfying and stellar side dishes, and in many cases will help you get the maximum nutrient benefits as well. In this section, we'll share several ways to cook vegetables to help you get the most enjoyment out of them during this stage and beyond.

Boiling and blanching: Boiling is one of the most common methods of cooking with liquid. It's also probably the number one cause of overcooked, soggy, and bland vegetables. Instead of boiling, we recommend that you try blanching vegetables. Similar to boiling, blanching involves cooking veggies in heated water, but you'll use a much shorter cooking time and then finish with a quick dip in ice water to stop the cooking process; this keeps vegetables crisp and bright and full of nutrients. You can blanch green beans, broccoli, cauliflower, asparagus, carrot sticks, sugar snap peas, and spinach. To blanch, simply bring a pot of lightly salted water to a boil and add your prepped veggies. Cook the veggies for 2 to 5 minutes depending on how al dente you like vegetables. While the veggies are cooking, prepare a bowl of ice water. Once the veggies are cooked, drain the water and toss your veggies into the ice bath for a few seconds to stop the cooking process. Enjoy as a side or snack, or add to salads.

Steaming: Steaming allows for vapors from a small amount of water to cook food. Steamed vegetables are likely to retain their vitamins and minerals since none of this goodness is lost to cooking liquid. Steaming could not be simpler: all you need is a large pot with a lid and a steamer basket. Cut fresh vegetables into small to medium uniform sizes (this helps them cook quickly and evenly). Add a small amount of water—one inch or less—to the bottom of your pot, and place the steamer basket on top, turning on the burner to high heat. Once the water is boiling or you begin to see steam, drop your prepped vegetables into the basket and top with a lid, lowering heat to medium. Cooking time will depend on the vegetable you're making—asparagus and broccoli will take just a few minutes, but firmer vegetables like carrots might require eight to ten minutes of cooking time. You can steam carrots, green beans, leafy greens, squash, and other tender vegetables. Adding aromatic spices, such as cinnamon sticks, lemongrass, or ginger, to the steaming liquid can infuse subtle, calorie-free flavors into your vegetables. See page 205 for more on steaming, including how to steam your favorite lean proteins.

Stir-frying: There are three ways to make sure you cook up great-tasting stir-fried vegetables: 1) prep all your ingredients into bite-size pieces before you begin, 2) make sure the veggies are dry so they're stir-fried and not steamed, and 3) use high heat. For cooking, use a wok, bowl-shaped skillet, or a large sauté pan. Don't use a nonstick-pan since it generally does not hold up over 500°F. Have a teaspoon of cooking oil—canola, peanut, or any other oil with a high smoke point—and a preportioned amount of low-sodium soy sauce, rice wine vinegar, or chicken broth ready (you might be tempted to use more oil, but be careful, as this can quickly add extra calories to an otherwise healthful dish). You can also prepare some minced garlic, chili peppers, or ginger if you'd like a bigger kick of flavor.

Heat the oil over high heat and add other cooking liquid such as low-sodium soy sauce. Stir in garlic, ginger, or peppers, if you're using them, and cook for about thirty seconds. Then, add your prepped veggies and cook for approximately five to seven minutes, depending on desired doneness.

If you're making a stir-fry dish with protein, such as chicken or beef, you may need to cook in batches. You can cook your protein selection first and then set it aside, using the same pan to then stir-fry your vegetables. Once the veggies are done, return the meat to the wok or sauté pan, and mix to bring the dish together.

Bell peppers, broccoli, carrots, mushrooms, onions, and sugar snap or snow peas are excellent when stir-fried (alone or as part of a main dish).

Roasting: You can bring out the best in many vegetables by roasting them. The high heat used in this cooking technique will bring out a vegetable's natural sweetness and in some cases add a little crunch. Prep vegetables in uniform sizes and shapes (as best you can) and spread onto a shallow baking pan in a single layer, leaving a little space between the pieces. Drizzle a slight amount (less than a teaspoon) of extra-virgin olive oil and a light sprinkle of kosher salt and pepper; toss to make sure all of the individual pieces are coated. Roast at 450°F for fifteen to twenty minutes or until you begin to see the edges of your veggies turn golden brown.

If vegetables are in season and roasted properly, you'll find that they don't need much more than light salt and pepper, but don't be afraid to experiment a little. Try fresh or dried herb and veggie combinations, such as thyme and broccoli, or add chopped garlic to the sheet pan before you start cooking. A squeeze of lemon juice or even zest can be a nice addition as well. When you get to Stage 3, you can top with a light dusting of Parmesan cheese for added flavor. Green beans, asparagus, cauliflower, broccoli, carrots, beets, and Brussels sprouts are all delicious when roasted.

Grilling: Just like with roasting, grilling locks in a vegetable's flavor, sometimes even adding a crispy sweetness. A big part of making great-tasting grilled vegetables is making sure your grill is clean. While the grill is heating up, clean the grate with a stiff wire brush, and then spray it with vegetable oil to prevent foods from sticking. Prepped veggies can get a light sprinkle of kosher salt and freshly ground pepper, and then should be placed on a hot grill, whether individually or in a grilling basket. Vegetables will be grilled anywhere from four to ten minutes total—you'll know they are done once they're golden and tender. Zucchini, squash, onions, asparagus, bell peppers, and mushrooms taste great when grilled. And once you get to Stage 7, you can add starchy vegetables such as corn and sweet potatoes to the grill as well.

Sautéing: Sautéing is a quick and easy way to cook veggies and is healthy as well since it usually requires relatively little oil for cooking (you can even sauté in water to avoid extra calories). As with most other cooking techniques, you'll want to slice, dice, or chop your vegetables into bite-size pieces so that they'll cook evenly and quickly. Heat a sauté pan over high heat, and then add 1 teaspoon of oil. Once the oil begins to shimmer—after a few seconds—add your vegetables. Lower heat to medium-high and toss until tender. Cooking time will depend on the desired tenderness and characteristics of the vegetables, but will typically range from five to ten minutes. Tender vegetables, such as asparagus, baby artichokes, snow peas, sweet peppers, onions, and mushrooms, are ideal for sautéing.

How Long to Follow Stage 2

You may stay on Stage 2 as long as you like since it is a healthful, complete, and balanced diet. As a general guideline, we suggest you add one week on this stage for every fifteen pounds you plan to lose. This means if you have thirty pounds to lose, you should follow Stage 2 for two weeks; sixty pounds to lose, four weeks, and so on. The goal is to get comfortable with the protein and vegetable structure of this meal plan, as these two foods will be the bulk of your meals for the rest of your life. Many of our most successful participants have stayed on Stage 2 for many weeks. They found that Stage 2 kept them fully satiated, that the simple structure of the meals made meal planning easy, and that their weight came off rapidly. Keep in mind that getting through these stages is not a race—you are working to create permanent changes, not just temporary fixes.

Dining Out During Stage 2 (and Beyond)

Dining out gets much easier in Stage 2. You can order a salad with dressing on the side plus all the nonstarchy vegetables you want. Be sure to order the vegetables steamed and without any added butter, oil, or sauces. If you order a salad as your main course, ask how much protein comes with the meal because it's important to continue to get 4 to 6 ounces of protein per meal to ensure you stay satiated. You can also still order a cup of berries for dessert, if you'd like. Follow these guidelines for any dining out you do during the remainder of the Seven Stages, or until you have reached your goal weight and have begun the maintenance plan.

Stage 2 Nutrition Summary

Since we're merely building upon the dietary changes you made in Stage 1, not much changes for you in Stage 2. Continue following the same caloric guidelines and eating the same foundational foods: proteins,

STAGE 2 NUTRITION SPECIFICS

Women: 1,100–1,400 calories per day
Men: 1,300–1,700 calories per day

BREAKFAST:	CALORIES	FAT (G)
4 ounces very lean protein	140	0–4
2 servings healthy fat (page 101)	90	10
1 cup berries	80	0
OR: 20/20 High Protein Dry Powder Breakfast Shake made with 1 cup berries and 1 tablespoon nut butter	360	10
OR: 20/20 High Protein Ready to Drink Breakfast Shake served with 1 cup berries and 1 tablespoon nut butter	309	14

LUNCH:	CALORIES	FAT (G)
WOMEN: 4 ounces very lean/lean protein	140–220	0–12
MEN: 6 ounces very lean/lean protein	210–330	0–18
1 serving healthy fat (for very lean protein only)	45	5
3 or more servings nonstarchy vegetables	45	0
1 cup berries	80	0

DINNER:	CALORIES	FAT (G)
WOMEN: 6 ounces very lean/lean protein	210-330	0–18
MEN: 8 ounces very lean/lean protein	280-440	0–24
1 serving healthy fat (for very lean protein only)	45	5
3 or more servings nonstarchy vegetables	45	0
1 cup berries	80	0

SNACK

WOMEN: 1 per day between lunch and dinner
MEN: 2 per day, 1 between breakfast and lunch, and 1 between lunch and dinner

Select one of these options per snack:	CALORIES	FAT (G)
2 ounces very lean protein + 1 cup berries	130	0–2
20/20 High Protein Dry Powder Breakfast Shake made with 1 cup berries (no nut butter)	260	0
20/20 High Protein Ready to Drink Breakfast Shake served with 1 cup berries (no nut butter)	220	6

healthy fats, and berries. The changes you make during Stage 2 will help you feel fuller and increase your vitamin, mineral, and nutrient intake:

- Eat six servings (three with lunch and three with dinner) of non-starchy vegetables each day. Nonstarchy vegetables include foods such as leafy greens, asparagus, carrots, zucchini, and broccoli.

- A serving of a nonstarchy vegetable (15 to 30 calories per serving), will vary based on type (see page 113 for full list):

    Leafy greens: 1 serving = 1½ cups
    Green vegetables: 1 serving = ½ cup
    Other nonstarchy vegetables: 1 serving = ½ cup

- Enjoy salad dressings, marinades, or sauces as your healthy fat. Select varieties that contain less than 6 grams of fat, 6 grams of sugar, and 400 milligrams of sodium per serving.

Stage 2 Exercise Plan: Maintaining Momentum

In the second stage of the Love Diet, your body might begin to protect itself against weight loss. It can do this by trying to hold on to stored calories (fat) or by lowering your level of non-exercise activity thermogenesis (NEAT), which is the calories you burn just by moving your body throughout the day, whether it's walking across the hall or fidgeting during a meeting. Keeping your NEAT caloric burn up during this stage is important to continuing your metabolic momentum. The easiest way to keep NEAT up is to make a conscious effort to reach five to six thousand steps per day on your pedometer. Remember, these are non-exercise steps! If you get home at the end of your day and find that your step count is below five thousand, get outside for a quick walk or even do laps inside your house if you have to—do whatever needs to be done to ensure that you hit your step goal. If you want to accelerate your weight loss, you can increase steps beyond the five to six thousand range; many of our successful participants increased their step goal to ten thousand each day.

For Stage 2, exercise will be as follows:

Level 1, Low Fitness: Moderate-speed walking 30 minutes, at least 5 days per week. Increase your pace to reach and maintain your minimum optimum heart rate,* which is 55 percent to 65 percent of your maximum heart rate.

---

* Remember: To figure out your optimum heart rate, take 220 and subtract your age, and then multiply the resulting number by 0.65; this equals the low end of your optimum heart rate. Next, take 220 and subtract your age, this time multiplying by 0.85; this equals the high end of your optimum heart rate. You can turn back to page 85 to see a sample calculation.

Level 2, Moderate Fitness: High-speed walking 30 minutes, running 5 minutes, at least 5 days per week. If running is difficult for you, continue high-speed walking for the additional 5 minutes. Keep your heart rate at the optimum level (between 65 percent and 85 percent of your maximum).

Level 3, High Fitness: Running 35 minutes, at least 5 days per week. Keep your heart rate at the optimum level.

All Levels: Reach at least 5,000 steps on your pedometer, excluding exercise.

Stage 2 Lifestyle Plan: Time Planning

As your body and mind become healthier, you will naturally become more efficient and productive, finding that you get more done in less time. If you still feel it's a struggle to fit everything into your life, it's important to step back and take stock of how you spend your time. Are you getting the most out of time spent, especially the minutes and hours you get to enjoy with the people most important to you? Sometimes you might feel that family time suffers when you make commitments to improve yourself, and yet the time invested will only make you a better partner, parent, and friend.

During this stage, we recommend becoming more conscious about the quality of the time you spend each day. Look at the time spent with your kids, significant others, friends, and family members and see how much of it includes staring at a screen, whether it's a TV, smartphone, or computer. When screens are present, we are naturally distracted and removed from the people in our presence. Suggest some screen-free plans by picking activities to do together that don't allow for the distraction—invite them to join you on your walk, check out a new hiking trail, play a board game, visit the batting cages, play miniature golf, or eat a picnic in the park. Remember, the Love Diet is all about positive, enriching transformations—don't be afraid to get out there and try new things!

CHAPTER 8

Stage 3: Protein Power

Welcome to Stage 3! By this point, you've discovered that combining proteins and veggies can satisfy your hunger and make it easier to lose those extra pounds. The good news is that with each stage you complete, your results will become even more noticeable and impressive.

You've also likely discovered how good it feels to care for yourself in a way that you had previously reserved for others. There's a very deep and rewarding satisfaction that comes from prepping and enjoying healthful meals and from following through with your commitments to yourself to exercise and eat according to plan. Each time you do this, you strengthen your self-acceptance and self-love skills by honoring the promises you've made to yourself. Remember, it takes practice!

Stage 3 features an eating plan that feels less like a diet and more like a long-term, maintainable way of eating. You may also follow Stage 3 as long as you like until you progress to the next stage. This stage highlights the addition of dairy-sourced proteins: low-fat cheese, low-fat or nonfat cottage cheese, and nonfat plain Greek yogurt (put a hold on the fruit-flavored yogurts until later in the eating plan). You can add up to two servings of these high-protein dairy foods to your meal plan each day. If your traditional diet does not include dairy, do not feel obligated to add it back in at this time; simply continue on Stage 2 for another week or go directly to Stage 4. If you've been anxiously awaiting the return of dairy, let's dig a little deeper into the foods you'll get to enjoy this week—we're confident you're going to love and appreciate the new dairy additions!

High-Protein Foods

All foods are made up of some combination of three macronutrients—carbohydrates, proteins, and fats. As you move forward through the stages of your meal plan, you will learn to classify foods by their greatest macronutrient percentage. For example, since nonfat plain Greek yogurt and low-fat versions of cheese contain more protein than fat or carbohydrates, they are classified throughout the Seven Stages as lean proteins (you can also think of them as dairy-sourced proteins).

When selecting dairy foods for Stage 3, be sure to refer to the nutrition label and make sure what you're getting has at least double the amount of protein grams to carbohydrate grams and less than 6 grams of fat per ounce. Here's an example of a nonfat plain Greek yogurt that would qualify as an acceptable Stage 3 dairy-sourced protein:

Nutrition Facts

Serving Size: 1 (1 Container; 170 grams)	
Amount Per Serving	
Calories 100	Calories from Fat 0
	% Daily Value
Total Fat 0 g	0%
Saturated Fat 0 g	0%
Trans Fat 0 g	
Cholesterol 10 mg	3%
Sodium 65 mg	3%
Total Carbohydrate 7 g	2%
Dietary Fiber 0 g	0%
Sugar 7 g	
Protein 18 g	36%

Your new protein foods won't be replacing any of the other foods you've been eating up until this point, but you will be making room for them by adjusting the portion size of your lean and very lean proteins so that you're still getting 4 to 8 ounces per serving (varies based on gender). We do this to keep your calorie intake in the range of 1,100 to 1,400 for women and 1,400 to 1,700 for men. You will continue to eat the same portions of healthy fats, berries, and nonstarchy vegetables as you did during Stage 2.

Making adjustments to your proteins is easy: you will just need to decrease your daily lean or very lean protein serving by 1 ounce and then add in a dairy protein to get the total amount of protein you need with each meal. For example, instead of 4 ounces of chicken, you can eat 3 ounces of chicken plus ¼ cup shredded cheese, which will bring you back up to 4 total ounces. For men, you will drop your lean or very lean protein portion down to 5 ounces instead of 6.

Your dairy protein servings will be as follows:

Low-fat cheese, shredded: 1 serving = 1 ounce or ¼ cup

Low-fat cheese, cubed or sliced: 1 serving = a slice the size of a Post-it Note or a cube the size of two dominoes

Nonfat plain Greek yogurt: 1 serving = ½ cup

Low-fat and nonfat cottage cheese: 1 serving = ¼ cup

Aim to include no more than two servings of dairy proteins per day. There are two reasons for this limitation: 1) each serving of dairy will provide you with 35 to 90 calories, which can add up quickly, and 2) dairy products, even low-fat and nonfat varieties, can sometimes slow or halt weight loss altogether.

Here are some of the recommended cheese, cottage cheese, and yogurt varieties to try during Stage 3:

Cheese

CHEDDAR

Trader Joe's Reduced Fat
Trader Joe's Sliced Lite
Trader Joe's Reduced Fat Celtic
Cabot Extra Light
Cabot Light

MOZZARELLA

Kraft 2% Shredded

STRING CHEESE

Frigo CheeseHeads Light (1 stick)
Kraft 2% (1 stick)
Sargento Light (1 stick)

SWISS

Jarlsberg Lite
Finlandia Light Swiss
Laughing Cow Creamy Swiss Light (2 wedges = 1 serving)
Laughing Cow Mini Babybel Light (1 round piece = 1 serving)
Kraft 2% (¾ ounce slice)

COLBY JACK

Kraft, Reduced Fat

PARMESAN

Kraft Reduced Fat Parmesan Style Grated Topping
(Use 2 tablespoons as a condiment for flavor)

FETA

Athenos Reduced Fat
President Fat Free Feta Crumbles

RICOTTA

Nonfat or low-fat varieties (¼ cup)

BRIE

Trader Joe's Light

BLUE CHEESE

Treasure Cave Reduced Fat Crumbled

Cottage Cheese

Fat-free or low-fat varieties (¼ cup)

High-Protein Yogurt

If you select yogurt from this list, be sure that the grams of protein are equal to or greater than twice the amount of carbohydrate grams.

Chobani Non-Fat Plain
Dannon Oikos Greek Nonfat Plain
Fage Total 0% Plain
Siggi's 0% Plain
Smári Pure Nonfat
Trader Joe's Greek Style 0% Nonfat Plain
Voskos Nonfat Plain

Bonus Strategies for Success

As you prepare to add new proteins this week, we have one piece of advice: be wary of dairy. It's been the undoing of many past dieters. If you follow our suggestions, you'll be able to enjoy increased variety in your meals and still continue to lose weight. Here's what we recommend to help you stay on track:

Measure carefully: It's easy to add on calories with dairy proteins, so pay extra attention to portions. A quarter cup of cheese should not be packed down, and servings of Greek yogurt or cottage cheese should be level and not heaping.

Get creative: Nonfat plain Greek yogurt will definitely hit your taste buds with a noticeable tang. If you don't like the tart flavor, don't just tolerate it; make it better! We recommend adding 1 cup of frozen thawed berries to ½ cup of Greek yogurt for your snack. You'll be amazed at how much the natural fruit sugars transform plain yogurt into a sweet and delectable treat. You can also add two light Laughing Cow wedges (one serving) to vegetables, or ¼ cup of low-fat shredded cheese to a salad. Another favorite is the lettuce burger: a grilled lean turkey burger and a 1-ounce slice of low-fat Swiss cheese with mustard or low-fat mayo, wrapped in lettuce. Don't be afraid to mix it up—this will help keep your palate interested in the process.

Mind the scale: As we mentioned, dairy can have a negative effect on weight loss for some people. For this reason, we recommend using the scale to monitor your progress. If you notice your weight loss slowing down or experience stomach discomfort, it could be due to the dairy proteins you've just added in. If this happens to you, remove all cheese, nonfat Greek yogurt, and low-fat and nonfat cottage cheese from your meals until you've reached your desired weight. Once you have reached your goal weight, you can add these items back in moderation. If you find that once again you gain weight or experience abdominal pain or bloating with the return of dairy, consider removing it from your diet altogether.

Stage 3 Nutrition Summary

This stage marks the return (or introduction) of select dairy proteins to your diet. Follow these serving guidelines to continue with your weight loss success:

Eat two or fewer servings of the following dairy proteins each day:

- Low-fat cheese, shredded: 1 serving = 1 ounce or ¼ cup
- Low-fat cheese, cubed or sliced: 1 serving = a slice the size of a Post-it Note or a cube the size of 2 dominoes
- Nonfat plain Greek yogurt: 1 serving = ½ cup
- Low-fat and nonfat cottage cheese: 1 serving = ¼ cup

When adding to a meal, make room for a serving of dairy protein by reducing the lean or very lean protein amount by 1 ounce.

Stage 3 Exercise Plan: Your Changing Body

Thanks to your dedication and hard work, your ligaments, tendons, muscles, and joints have grown stronger over the last two stages. This will allow for greater increases in intensity, which will improve your fitness and further charge your rebalanced metabolism.

Be sure to check in with your body after exercise. It's normal to feel a little sore for a day or so, but you shouldn't be experiencing chronic soreness. If your muscle soreness doesn't seem to go away, look to your

STAGE 3 NUTRITION SPECIFICS

Women: 1,100–1,400 calories per day
Men: 1,300–1,700 calories per day

BREAKFAST:	CALORIES	FAT (G)
4 ounces very lean protein	140	0–4
2 servings healthy fat (page 101)	90	10
1 cup berries	80	0
OR: 20/20 High Protein Dry Powder Breakfast Shake made with 1 cup berries and 1 tablespoon nut butter	360	10
OR: 20/20 High Protein Ready to Drink Breakfast Shake served with 1 cup berries and 1 tablespoon nut butter	309	14

LUNCH:	CALORIES	FAT (G)
WOMEN: 4 ounces very lean/lean protein	140–220	0–12
OR: 3 ounces very lean/lean protein + 1 ounce cheese		
MEN: 6 ounces very lean/lean protein	210–330	0–18
OR: 5 ounces very lean/lean protein + 1 ounce cheese		
1 serving healthy fat (for very lean protein only)	45	5
3 or more servings nonstarchy vegetables	45	0
1 cup berries	80	0

DINNER:	CALORIES	FAT (G)
WOMEN: 6 ounces very lean/lean protein	210–330	0–18
OR: 5 ounces very lean/lean protein + 1 ounce cheese		
MEN: 8 ounces very lean/lean protein	280–440	0–24
OR: 7 ounces very lean/lean protein + 1 ounce cheese		
1 serving healthy fat (for very lean protein only)	45	5
3 or more servings nonstarchy vegetables	45	0
1 cup berries	80	0

SNACK

WOMEN: 1 per day between lunch and dinner

MEN: 2 per day, 1 between breakfast and lunch and 1 between lunch and dinner

Note: If your snack contains two dairy servings, then this would complete your dairy limit for the day

Select one of these options per snack:	CALORIES	FAT (G)
½ cup nonfat/low-fat plain Greek yogurt + 1 cup berries	130–150	0–2
2 low-fat string cheese sticks + 1 cup berries	180–200	5
2 ounces very lean protein + 1 cup berries	130	0–2
20/20 High Protein Dry Powder Breakfast Shake made with 1 cup berries (no nut butter)	260	0
20/20 High Protein Ready to Drink Breakfast Shake served with 1 cup berries (no nut butter)	220	6

sleep habits for clues. Are you sleeping at least seven and a half hours a night? You need adequate rest to help your body fully recover and repair itself after exercise.

During this stage, you will want to increase your pedometer steps to a minimum of six thousand steps per day, making sure to record daily steps in your tracker. You can increase your steps by always looking for the on-foot option. Instead of getting on the elevator, try taking the stairs, or park on the far side of the parking lot and watch the extra steps accumulate as you walk to the office or store. If you have a sedentary job, try to get up once an hour for a two-minute break—head to the cooler for some hydration or just do a quick lap around the space if you can.

For Stage 3, exercise will be as follows:

Level 1, Low Fitness: Moderate to high-speed walking 45 minutes, at least 5 days per week. Aim to reach and maintain your minimum optimum heart rate (65 percent of your maximum).

Level 2, Moderate Fitness: High-speed walking 30 minutes, running 15 minutes, at least 5 days per week. If running is difficult for you, add an extra 15 minutes of high-speed walking, preferably on gradual hills to keep your heart rate up. Maintain an intensity that allows you to achieve your optimum heart rate (between 65 percent and 85 percent of your maximum).

Level 3, High Fitness: Running 45 minutes, at least 5 days per week. Add gradual hills to increase intensity. Maintain your optimum heart rate (between 65 percent and 85 percent of your maximum).

All Levels: Take at least 6,000 steps per day, not including exercise.

Stage 3 Lifestyle Plan: Checking In on Sleep and Stress

During this stage, we recommend paying special attention to how you're responding to stress and how much sleep you're getting (seven and a half to eight and a half hours a night is ideal). Even if you think you're immune to the effects of too little sleep or too much stress, we challenge you to track levels of sleep and stress to see how they impact your results and your overall quality of life. We often have people who come into the clinic who are oblivious of, or in denial about, the toll that poor sleep or excess stress takes on their lives. Yet when they make an effort to increase or improve sleep and manage stress better, they experience a noticeable boost in well-being, an increase in energy levels, and accelerated weight loss. This was especially true for Arthur, who came to us at 20/20 LifeStyles when he was twenty-five, already seventy pounds overweight, ready to change his life.

Before Arthur came to us, he thought of himself as bulletproof. He was still living life the way he and his college buddies used to—burning the candle at both ends, using and abusing his body. And yet he knew his chronic lack of sleep (two to four hours a night), late-night meals, and nearly constant intake of caffeine and nicotine were catching up with him and likely to blame for his poor mental and physical health—besides being overweight, he had high blood pressure and very high cholesterol and was chronically depressed. Arthur tried catching up on sleep during the weekends, sometimes sleeping as much as ten hours a day, but he still felt miserable most of the time. He had tried to change his behavior and his lifestyle before, hiring a personal trainer and using smoking cessation programs, but nothing seemed to work.

It wasn't until he learned to expand his definition of *lifestyle* that he was able to change his life. He had to consider not just exercise and his smoking habits but his sleeping habits, eating habits, and stress levels as well. Through 20/20 LifeStyles, Arthur discovered that he was chemically and metabolically imbalanced due to cigarettes, soda, lack of sleep, and poor food choices, and that he would have to make changes in these habits to improve his health. When it came down to it, the modifications he made in those areas were critical to his success, but he found the mental changes he made were equally as important.

When Arthur learned to love himself, he found that he intuitively didn't want to hurt his body anymore. He had never considered how important self-respect and self-love were to his health, but he learned that telling himself he was worth it made all the difference in finally becoming happy and healthy.

Arthur went on to lose sixty-nine pounds and no longer has high cholesterol or high blood pressure. He corrected his sleeping habits, learned to manage his stress better, followed the Seven Stages, and began exercising at least five times a week.

You, too, can make improvements to your sleep and stress management skills; even just small changes can produce benefits relatively quickly. Start with a goal to get to bed five minutes earlier than usual, or try to carve out a few minutes in the morning to meditate, and then build from there. If you can commit to these habits, you will experience unexpected rewards—you will feel an increase in calm and peace of mind, and you will find that making decisions and handling a busy schedule will become easier. You will feel more motivated to exercise and stay on top of your new eating habits.

For additional sleep and stress management strategies, including more on the incredible benefits of meditation and how to get started, visit the Resources section.

CHAPTER 9

Stage 4: Favorite Fruits

Congratulations on reaching Stage 4! By now, you could be down two pant or dress sizes or have found yourself needing a much tighter belt. And there's no doubt that you're experiencing renewed energy and confidence in yourself. You should be proud of the changes you've made as well as the outpouring of love you've directed your own way—you deserve it.

We're going to continue to guide you down the path to permanent weight loss, and we couldn't be prouder of the progress you've made so far. Now is a good time to check in with your positive visualization practices—are you working through any potentially tough situations in your head first? Are you using visualization for motivation, envisioning yourself weeks or months from now doing activities you haven't done in years? Your mind is very powerful—use it to help make success easier!

In Stage 4, you will be reintroducing all fruits to your diet. Berries have carried you this far and have done a lot to satisfy your needs and cravings for carbs; plus, they've also been a big help in restoring balance to your blood sugar. But we bet you're ready to bring some other delicious fruit flavors into your diet!

The key to Stage 4 is awareness of portion sizes. Because berries are considered a safe carb, you were able to (and still can) enjoy a 1 cup serving size of raspberries, blueberries, blackberries, and other berries. Other fruits, however, will have higher levels of carbohydrates, so those with higher amounts will be offered in a ½ cup serving size. Remember, a greater percentage of simple carbohydrates in a food can result in a quicker absorption of sugar in the body. This could cause you to experience hunger and cravings. Apples, pears, and oranges will have a serving the size of a tennis ball, and fruits such as grapes, melon, and pineapple will have a serving size of ½ cup (level, not heaping). An easy way to remember fruit serving sizes is to think of this phrase: *Berries are good; you can have twice as many. For the rest of the fruits, a half cup is plenty!*

Your fruit serving sizes will be as follows:

1 serving of non-berry fruit = ½ cup

1 serving of berries = 1 cup

Whole fruits: 1 serving = 1 medium fruit (equal to the size of a tennis ball)

Here are some fruits that we recommend:

Apple
Apricot
Banana (½ medium)
Blackberries
Blueberries
Boysenberries
Cantaloupe
Cherries
Grapefruit
Grapes
Honeydew melon
Kiwifruit
Mango
Marionberries
Nectarine
Orange
Papaya
Peach
Pear
Pineapple
Plums
Raspberries
Strawberries
Tangerines
Watermelon

Three Simple Ways to Make Fruit More Satiating

Keeping your non-berry fruit servings in check will help prevent the type of blood sugar spikes that lead to subsequent crashes and intense cravings. Here are a few other strategies for enjoying fruit without negatively affecting your hunger and weight loss:

Always eat fruit with a protein or fat source: Protein and healthy fats break down in your body slower than carbohydrates, and smart combinations of these foods will keep you feeling satisfied between meals. Pair one serving of fruit with two servings of a healthy fat or 2 ounces of protein; this will give you a perfectly balanced snack with a 1:1 carbohydrate to protein ratio.

Some of our favorite healthy fats to pair with a serving of fruit are 1 tablespoon of nut butter, 12 almonds, or ¼ of an avocado. Proteins include items such as 2 low-fat string cheese sticks or 2 ounces low-sodium deli meat. A perfect pair might be one tennis ball–size apple (carbohydrate) eaten with ½ cup low-fat cottage cheese (protein).

Apply this rule to all carbohydrates. Never eat a carb alone! For blood sugar control, a carbohydrate should always be paired with a protein or healthy fat.

Pick frozen fruits wisely: When using frozen fruits, always choose the unsweetened variety. Added sweeteners can increase the amount of sugar and bump up the calorie content significantly. Sweetened fruits are also more likely to send your blood sugar sky-high.

Avoid dried fruits and fruit juices: Dried fruit provides more calories and less volume than whole fruit. For example, ½ cup of raisins (dried grapes) equals 220 calories, while a ½ cup of grapes is just 60 calories. And fruit juices provide too many nonsatiating calories. Instead of drinking fruit juice, eat whole, fresh fruits. One delicious, juicy orange, the size of a tennis ball, is just 60 calories and you'll get 3 grams of filling fiber too. The fruit juice equivalent of 60 calories is just ½ cup, which will provide only ½ gram of fiber. Whole fruit wins every time!

Monitor your fruit response: Some fruits may make you hungrier than others. If you add back in a certain fruit and find that it triggers intense hunger or cravings, take it back out of your diet.

As we've mentioned, your body can get sufficient carbohydrates from berries; if you notice cravings with all other fruits, return to eating your 1 cup serving of berries with meals.

Stage 4 Nutrition Summary

This stage is all about enjoying a wider variety of colorful fruits. You will also notice that in Stage 4 and subsequent stages, the protein amount during your dinner decreases. This is designed to keep your calories in an optimal range as you add back the different food groups. Stay in Stage 4 for as long as you like before you progress to Stage 5. Follow these guidelines with fruit to ensure you continue to promote weight loss and maintain balanced blood sugar:

- Enjoy two to four servings of fruits, which now includes non-berry fruits, each day; specific serving sizes are as follows:

  Small or cut fruits: 1 serving = ½ cup
  Berries: 1 serving = 1 cup
  Whole fruits: 1 serving = one medium fruit (the size of a tennis ball)

- For best results, pair one fruit serving with two servings of a healthy fat or 2 ounces of protein, e.g., one small apple with 1 tablespoon nut butter.

Stage 4 Exercise Plan: Redefining Your Limits

You're at the point now where you're just beginning to recognize your potential with exercise. You're starting to push aside the self-imposed mental barriers and do things you never thought possible. We encourage you to continue using your heart rate monitor as a measurement—you are growing stronger, fitter, and healthier every day, and your potential is growing in response to these improvements. Keep going!

STAGE 4 NUTRITION SPECIFICS

Women: 1,100–1,400 calories per day
Men: 1,300–1,700 calories per day

BREAKFAST:	CALORIES	FAT (G)
4 ounces very lean protein	140	0–4
2 servings healthy fat (page 101)	90	10
½ cup fruit or 1 cup berries	60–80	0
OR: 20/20 High Protein Dry Powder Breakfast Shake made with 1 cup berries and 1 tablespoon nut butter	360	10
OR: 20/20 High Protein Ready to Drink Breakfast Shake served with 1 cup berries and 1 tablespoon nut butter	309	14

LUNCH:	CALORIES	FAT (G)
WOMEN: 4 ounces very lean/lean protein	140–220	0–12
OR: 3 ounces very lean/lean protein + 1 ounce cheese		
MEN: 6 ounces very lean/lean protein	210–330	0–18
OR: 5 ounces very lean/lean protein + 1 ounce cheese		
1 serving healthy fat (for very lean protein only)	45	5
3 or more servings of nonstarchy vegetables	45	0
½ cup fruit	60	0
OR: 1 cup berries	80	0

DINNER:	CALORIES	FAT (G)
WOMEN: 4 ounces very lean/lean protein	140–220	0–12
OR: 3 ounces very lean/lean protein + 1 ounce cheese		
MEN: 6 ounces very lean/lean protein	210–330	0–18
OR: 5 ounces very lean/lean protein + 1 ounce cheese		
1 serving healthy fat (for very lean protein only)	45	5
3 or more servings of nonstarchy vegetables	45	0
½ cup fruit	60	0
OR: 1 cup berries	80	0

SNACK

WOMEN: 1 per day between lunch and dinner
MEN: 2 per day, 1 between breakfast and lunch, and 1 between lunch and dinner

Select one of these options per snack:	CALORIES	FAT (G)
½ cup nonfat or low-fat cottage cheese + ½ cup fruit	160–180	0–2
½ cup nonfat or low-fat plain Greek yogurt + ½ cup fruit	140–170	0–4
2 ounces very lean protein + 1 cup berries	130	0–2
20/20 High Protein Dry Powder Breakfast Shake made with 1 cup berries (no nut butter)	260	0
20/20 High Protein Ready to Drink Breakfast Shake served with 1 cup berries (no nut butter)	220	6

Part of redefining your limits involves exploring sports and activities that are new to you. Have you tried racquetball, squash, skiing, hiking, or bicycling? Now might be the time to try something out of your comfort zone. You don't have to be a pro on the first try; the goal is to find additional activities you enjoy doing. Consider taking a lesson in something you've always wanted to try, and bring your family or friends along with you. Engaging in a new activity together can be a bonding experience and an opportunity for laughter, fun, and fitness—the perfect combination!

If you can't think of a new sport you'd like to try, check out the class list at your gym and peek in on one that interests you. There is endless variety in gym classes these days—whether you like strength training, dance, yoga, or cycling, you can find a class that suits you. If you find an activity that allows you to keep your heart rate at its optimum level, you can substitute this workout for one or more of your walking or running workouts.

For Stage 4, exercise will be as follows:

Level 1, Low Fitness: Your goal this stage is to incorporate some running into your workouts (if you can). High-speed walking 40 minutes, running 5 minutes, at least 5 days per week. If running is difficult for you, add an additional 5 minutes of high-speed walking instead of the run, preferably up a gradual hill to keep your heart rate high. Keep your pace at a level that allows you to stay at your optimum heart rate (between 65 percent and 85 percent of your maximum).

Level 2, Moderate Fitness: It's time to introduce interval training to your workouts. Instead of maintaining one level of intensity throughout a workout, you will now alternate between high and moderate intensity. This will increase your weight loss, strength, and endurance. Your Stage 4 interval session will be as follows:

10 minutes of high-speed walking
10 minutes of running or hill walking
10 minutes of high-speed walking (second set)
15 minutes of running or hill walking

Complete this workout at least 5 days per week, making sure to keep your heart rate at optimum level.

Level 3, High Fitness: Running 45 minutes, at least 5 days per week. Continue running gradual hills and keeping your heart rate at optimum level. You might consider starting to pay attention to your pace, which will give you a new goal to pursue—we suggest working toward being able to run a 10-minute mile. There are several free apps available that will allow you to track your runs and give you plenty of data, including your pace, time, distance, and even elevation. You could also find a park or walkway that has mile markers—check your watch when you begin a mile and again when you complete it. Identifying your personal starting pace is not about labeling yourself fast or slow, but instead about helping you establish a baseline that you can improve upon.

All Levels: Continue to wear a pedometer each day, aiming to reach at least 6,000 steps per day, excluding exercise.

Stage 4 Lifestyle Plan: To Lapse Is Human

When you first began the Seven Stages, you probably stayed clear of restaurants, dishes, or social situations that could trigger your overeating habits, and avoided certain diet assassins in your life—people who sabotage your efforts to eat well and exercise more. But at this point in the plan, you have likely found that you're more willing to test yourself, even in the face of challenging situations. While it's important to test yourself because it's truly the only way to continue to strengthen your ability to stick to healthy eating habits, it's also important to note that taking on greater challenges can present a greater risk of slipups. And when—not if—a slipup happens, you have to know how to respond in the most compassionate, constructive way possible.

When you slip up or lapse, turn your attention immediately to your self-talk and be sure to shut off any self-defeating statements. You can take charge of the tone by accepting responsibility, developing awareness of what specifically led you to fall off track, and then establishing a plan for how you'll handle the situation next time. Let's say you gave in to a tray of unhealthy appetizers at a party—your strategy for the next time could be to make sure that you've eaten before an event where there will be food.

When you respond constructively, you grant yourself the space and patience to grow into your new habits and you avoid the spiral into negative self-talk. Once you've reached the maintenance stage, your response to slipups will become especially important—which is why we go further into the discussion of lapses and relapses there (starting on page 173).

It's important to note that if you do lapse, your first response should be to review your meal tracker for that day and the previous two days. Ask yourself:

Have I been tracking within 15 minutes of eating?

Have I been eating my recommended amounts of protein and healthy fats?

Am I drinking enough water?

Have I added any new foods to my diet that may have caused cravings?

Have I been getting adequate sleep?

Have my stress levels changed?

The answers to these questions will often reveal the clues to why a lapse has occurred and help you get right back on track.

CHAPTER 10

Stage 5: Dairy Delights

In Stage 5, you will be reintroducing new types of dairy to your diet, including skim milk, low-fat milk, fruit-flavored yogurt, and fruit-flavored Greek yogurt. These foods are not a required part of your meal plan and can be left out if you've identified a dairy sensitivity or negative response (such as weight gain). While we've selected dairy options that will continue to promote metabolic balance and weight loss, be sure you're not turning to these foods in times of stress or strong emotion.

If you're ready to add these foods back in, let's show you how it's done.

The New Dairy Rules

The dairy-based foods you added during Stage 3 were all considered proteins because they provide a significant amount of protein in the makeup of their macronutrients. The dairy items you will reintroduce in this stage have varying macronutrient profiles that require different classifications. Non-Greek yogurts and skim and 1% milk are called carbohydrate-dominant dairy foods, meaning they have more carbs than protein, and are categorized as carbohydrates for this plan. Fruit-flavored Greek yogurts, which have nearly equal parts protein and carbohydrate, are considered a hybrid.

You will want to use nutrition labels to tell you how to classify dairy items, or select from our list of approved options. Here's an easy reference chart to help you remember which dairy foods fall into which category:

DAIRY PROTEINS (STAGE 3)

Low-fat cheese

Nonfat plain Greek yogurt

Low-fat and nonfat cottage cheese

DAIRY CARBS (STAGE 5)

All non-Greek yogurts

Skim milk

1% milk

DAIRY PROTEIN-CARB HYBRIDS (STAGE 5)

Fruit-flavored Greek yogurts

You can eat up to two servings per day of all dairy-based products; each serving will provide between 60 and 120 calories (this is the same for both men and women). Serving sizes are as follows:

1% or skim milk: 1 serving = 1 cup

Plain and fruit-flavored non-Greek yogurt: 1 serving = ½ cup

Plain and fruit-flavored Greek yogurt: 1 serving = ½ cup

Fruit-flavored Greek yogurt can be an ideal snack: it contains probiotics, which are good bacteria that can promote healthy digestion and boost immune strength, is satiating, and is relatively convenient and quick.

It's important to be selective with non-Greek yogurt, as certain varieties can have excess sugar and calories. When selecting non-Greek yogurts, make sure they meet these criteria:

Per ½ cup serving (4.32 ounces), yogurt should have:

130 calories or less

16 grams of sugar or less

No more than 25 grams of carbohydrates per 7 grams of protein

STALLED WEIGHT LOSS: IS DAIRY TO BLAME?

If you notice your weight loss begin to lag during this stage, keep a close eye on your dairy intake. Remember, if your snack contains 2 dairy servings, this completes your dairy limit for the day. Many people have trouble digesting lactose, the type of sugar found in milk and other dairy foods, leading to digestive distress. This doesn't mean you shouldn't include dairy in your diet; just know that it's one of the first places you should look if your weight loss slows.

To make it easy for you, we've selected a handful of widely available yogurts that you can enjoy during this stage:

CARBOHYDRATE YOGURTS

Cascade Fresh
Nancy's
Rachel's
Stonyfield
Wallaby
Yami

HYBRID YOGURTS

Dannon Oikos Greek Nonfat flavored
Chobani Greek Non-Fat flavored
Fage Total 0% Split Cup
Siggi's 0% flavored
Smári Nonfat flavored
Trader Joe's Greek Style 0% Nonfat flavored
Voskos Nonfat Greek flavored

Stage 5 Nutrition Summary

New dairy items hit the menu in this stage: low-fat milk, skim milk, fruit-flavored yogurt, and fruit-flavored Greek yogurt are now yours to enjoy.

- Eat up to 2 servings of these foods per day, with specific servings as follows:

  1% or skim milk: 1 serving = 1 cup
  Plain and fruit-flavored non-Greek yogurt: 1 serving = ½ cup
  Plain and fruit-flavored Greek yogurt: 1 serving = ½ cup

- Non-Greek yogurts, skim milk, and low-fat milk have more carbohydrates than protein and are therefore classified as carbohydrates. This expands your lunch and dinner carbohydrate options, which are now: berries, nonfat or low-fat flavored yogurt, or nonfat or low-fat milk.

STAGE 5 NUTRITION SPECIFICS

Women: 1,100–1,400 calories per day
Men: 1,300–1,700 calories per day

BREAKFAST:	CALORIES	FAT (G)
4 ounces very lean protein	140	0–4
2 servings healthy fat (page 101)	90	10
½ cup fruit or 1 cup berries	60–80	0
OR: 20/20 High Protein Dry Powder Breakfast Shake made with 1 cup berries and 1 tablespoon nut butter	360	10
OR: 20/20 High Protein Ready to Drink Breakfast Shake served with 1 cup berries and 1 tablespoon nut butter	309	14

LUNCH:	CALORIES	FAT (G)
WOMEN: 4 ounces very lean/lean protein	140–220	0–12
OR: 3 ounces very lean/lean protein + 1 ounce cheese		
MEN: 6 ounces very lean/lean protein	210–330	0–18
OR: 5 ounces very lean/lean protein + 1 ounce cheese		
1 serving healthy fat (for very lean protein only)	45	5
3 or more servings nonstarchy vegetables	45	0
Choose one of the carbohydrate choices listed below:	60–100	0–3
1 cup berries		
½ cup fruit		
½ cup nonfat or low-fat flavored yogurt		
1 cup nonfat or low-fat milk		

Stage 5 Exercise Plan: Look At Me!

Chances are that you used to see very fit people and think that they were different from you, part of a group to which you would never belong. But things have changed, and you have begun to see these people instead as individuals with whom you share common interests—namely, a healthy and active lifestyle. With each day of exercise, you open your world up a bit further as new opportunities begin to present themselves. You might be starting to hear questions like, "Do you want to be a chaperone on the kids' hiking trip next month?" "Are you interested in joining us for a bike ride?" "We need another player on our rec softball team—do you want to play?"

DINNER:	CALORIES	FAT (G)
WOMEN: 4 ounces very lean/lean protein	140–220	0–12
OR: 3 ounces very lean/lean protein + 1 ounce cheese		
MEN: 6 ounces very lean/lean protein	210–330	0–18
OR: 5 ounces very lean/lean protein + 1 ounce cheese		
1 serving healthy fat (for very lean protein only)	45	5
3 or more servings of nonstarchy vegetables	45	0
Choose one of the carbohydrate choices listed below:	60–100	0–3
1 cup berries		
½ cup fruit		
½ cup nonfat or low-fat flavored yogurt		
1 cup nonfat or low-fat milk		

SNACK

WOMEN: 1 per day between lunch and dinner

MEN: 2 per day, 1 between breakfast and lunch, and 1 between lunch and dinner

Select one of these options per snack:	CALORIES	FAT (G)
½ cup nonfat flavored Greek yogurt + 1–2 tablespoons nuts or seeds	140–220	5–10
¼ cup nonfat or low-fat cottage cheese + ½ cup nonfat or low-fat flavored yogurt	190–220	0–4
2 ounces very lean protein + 1 cup berries	130	0–2
20/20 High Protein Dry Powder Breakfast Shake made with 1 cup berries (no nut butter)	260	0
20/20 High Protein Ready to Drink Breakfast Shake served with 1 cup berries (no nut butter)	220	6

Of course, you don't have to wait for these types of questions to come to you—you can make it known to your friends and family that you're feeling great and are always open to participating in new and fun activities. Most importantly, the fear you used to have about missing out because of your weight or health should be fading—don't be afraid to let it go.

Before you dig into your exercise guidelines for this stage, take a moment to acknowledge the personal growth and progress you've made so far by following the Seven Stages—we have no doubt that you've already made an impressive transformation!

For Stage 5, exercise will be as follows:

Level 1, Low Fitness: High-speed walking 10 minutes, plus running or hill walking 5 minutes. Repeat this three times in a row, completing a total of 45 minutes of exercise. Perform at least 5 days per week. Your pace should be such that you reach your optimum heart rate (between 65 percent and 85 percent of your maximum).

Level 2, Moderate Fitness: High-speed walking 12 minutes, running or hill walking 20 minutes, and then high-speed walking for 12 minutes, at least 5 days per week. Keep your heart rate at optimum level (between 65 and 85 percent of your maximum).

Level 3, High Fitness: Running 45 minutes, at least 5 days per week. Continue running gradual hills and monitoring your pace. Maintain a pace that allows you to keep your heart rate at optimum level. Your goal is to work toward completing 6 miles in 60 minutes or better.

All Levels: Continue to wear your pedometer and record a minimum of 6,000 steps per day, excluding exercise.

Stage 5 Lifestyle Plan: The Truth Tablet

Part of becoming more grounded in the renewed sense of love and acceptance you have for yourself is knowing how to make decisions with confidence and without the influence of any lingering codependent behaviors. You might recall the truth test (see page 49), the mental exercise we taught you to use to help take the power out of self-defeating statements. We teach a similar technique for restoring decision-making confidence, called the Truth Tablet.

A Truth Tablet is essentially a pros-and-cons list that allows you to consider a decision from every angle. The most important part of completing a Truth Tablet is that it must be written down—writing can help you make difficult decisions because it gives you the ability to truly see all the factors involved. Here's how to complete your own.

At the top of a page of paper, write down the decision that's on your plate. Below that, write your two or three options, and under each option write *Advantages* and *Disadvantages*, leaving some space in between the words so you can begin to form vertical rows below. It should look something like this:

SHOULD I TAKE THE JOB OFFER FROM A NEW COMPANY?

Take offer		Stay at current job	
Advantage	**Disadvantage**	**Advantage**	**Disadvantage**
15% more money	Have to prove myself again	Respected here	Less money
Manager position	Don't know staff	May be manager soon	Unsure of promotion
A new challenge	Kids change school	Little stress	A bit bored at work

Once you have all the information laid out, read through it to see if a clear choice stands out. You can also share your Truth Tablet with a trusted friend, family member, or advisor and consider what they have to say. Remember to evaluate this from a place of confidence and aim to make decisions based on what's right for you, not for others. This doesn't mean you're being selfish, but it does mean that you're learning how to practice self-care.

CHAPTER 11

Stage 6: Legume Love

In Stage 6, you will be adding beans, lentils, and split peas back to your diet. These foods are legumes, which are the edible fruits or seeds that come from the shell or pod of a plant. Legumes contain a small amount of protein but typically have two to three times more carbohydrate content than protein, which is why we classify them as a carbohydrate. Follow Stage 6 until you are ready to progress to Stage 7.

You know what's great about legumes? Pretty much everything. They're inexpensive, satiating, and full of minerals, nutrients, and fiber. The only catch with legumes is that they are calorie-rich foods—since you are still working to promote weight loss, you will want to be smart about monitoring their portion sizes.

We recommend that you eat a ½ cup serving (about 100 calories) of beans, lentils, or split peas no more than twice a day, and only one serving per meal. In this meal, your serving of beans, lentils, or split peas would replace the previous serving of berries, fruit, or dairy that was there before. When you consider that a typical side of beans served at a Mexican restaurant is more than double this serving, you can see why it's important to pay attention to the portions you eat.

If you don't like beans, you don't have to eat them at this point or at all during the remaining stages. When you add carbohydrates to your meals while following this plan, it's important that they be carbs that you enjoy—as long as they are from the list of approved carbs, of course! Our goal with the Seven Stages is to rebuild your diet so it's sustainable and satisfying for you long term. Feel free to omit anything that doesn't suit your palate or body as long as you continue to consume enough calories. If you notice that legumes increase your hunger, stall weight loss, or lead to any digestive discomfort, you can remove them from your meal plan.

Say Hello to Hummus

Introducing beans to your diet in Stage 6 also means the return of hummus. If you haven't tried hummus, you are in for a treat; if you have, I'm sure you are happy to have it back. Hummus is a dip or spread made from pureed garbanzo beans, tahini or sesame paste, and extra-virgin olive oil. While it is mostly a carbohydrate, it also contains healthy fat and a little bit of protein, which makes it more of a hybrid food. Because it contains some fat and protein on its own, pairing it with a separate protein is optional.

As with other legumes and legume-based foods, you will want to carefully measure portions of hummus. You can consume a maximum of 2 to 4 level tablespoons per serving. The hybrid nature of hummus makes it a great stand-alone snack, but you can also pair it with 2 ounces of sliced lean turkey or raw sliced bell peppers—the latter is a perfect midafternoon Mediterranean snack that will tide you over until dinner. This smart snack provides you with 12 grams of protein, 6 grams of carbohydrates, and 4 grams of fat, all for just 110 calories.

Tips for Buying, Cooking, and Eating Beans

Cooking your own beans is easy—in most cases, you just buy dried beans, soak them overnight, and then simmer in water for a little over an hour or so, adding a pinch of salt when they're nearly done. When you make beans this way, you control the amount of salt in them. The other option is to buy canned beans, which are quicker and easier, but some varieties may provide more sodium than what you need. Follow these two tips to ensure that enjoying beans doesn't also mean exceeding the recommended amount of sodium each day:

- Buy only canned beans that say either *low sodium* or *no sodium* on the label. *Low sodium* should mean less than 400 mg per ½ cup serving.
- No matter what type of bean you buy, be sure to rinse them for one minute before using in a dish or eating directly. Rinsing them will decrease the sodium content by nearly 25 percent.

Beans are incredible flavor sponges and can add heartiness to otherwise light dishes. They make a great base for chili (see recipes on pages 226 and 227), increase a salad's satiety—simply add a serving of beans to any greens—and can easily be transformed into a tasty side. Add these seasonings and flavor boosters to make beans more satisfying:

- Hot peppers, garlic, and cilantro for Mexican flavor
- Garlic, oregano, basil, sage, and rosemary for an Italian kick
- Curry, turmeric, cumin, coriander, cayenne pepper, and ginger for Indian spice
- Diced vegetables, such as bell peppers, green or red onions, to increase a bean dish's freshness
- A bit of your favorite salsa
- High-protein nonfat Greek yogurt as a sour cream substitute
- ⅛ of an avocado for a serving of healthy fat

Here are some recommended varieties of beans you can try during Stage 6:

- Low-Sodium Canned Beans:
    - Bush's Low Sodium
    - Eden Organic
    - Westbrae Natural
    - Progresso
    - S&W 50% Less Sodium
- Refried Beans:
    - Rosarita No Fat

Stage 6 Nutrition Summary

You can enjoy all varieties of beans, lentils, split peas, and hummus in this stage. Remember, when you add beans to your meal, they count as your carbohydrate serving for that meal. The recommended serving sizes are as follows:

Cooked beans, lentils, and split peas: 1 serving = ½ cup (100 calories)

Hummus: 2–4 level tablespoons (100 calories total)

Aim to have no more than two servings of these carbohydrate foods per day.

STAGE 6 NUTRITION SPECIFICS

Women: 1,100–1,400 calories per day
Men: 1,300–1,700 calories per day

BREAKFAST:	CALORIES	FAT (G)
4 ounces very lean protein	140	0–4
2 servings healthy fat (page 101)	90	10
½ cup fruit or 1 cup berries	60–80	0
OR: 20/20 High Protein Dry Powder Breakfast Shake made with 1 cup berries and 1 tablespoon nut butter	360	10
OR: 20/20 High Protein Ready to Drink Breakfast Shake served with 1 cup berries and 1 tablespoon nut butter	309	14

LUNCH:	CALORIES	FAT (G)
WOMEN: 4 ounces very lean/lean protein	140–220	0–12
OR: 3 ounces very lean/lean protein + 1 ounce cheese		
MEN: 6 ounces very lean/lean protein	210–330	0–18
OR: 5 ounces very lean/lean protein + 1 ounce cheese		
1 serving healthy fat (for very lean protein)	45	5
3 or more servings nonstarchy vegetables	45	0
Choose one of the carbohydrate choices listed below:	60–100	0–3
1 cup berries		
½ cup fruit		
½ cup nonfat or low-fat flavored yogurt		
1 cup nonfat or low-fat milk		
½ cup cooked beans		

Stage 6 Exercise Plan: The Best Medicine of All

If you've been consistent with exercise throughout the Seven Stages, it's likely that with your doctor's guidance you've been able to remove some, if not all, medications from your life. Research has shown that exercise is as effective as medication in the treatment of conditions such as prediabetes, type 2 diabetes, and heart disease and the associated risk factors such as high cholesterol and high blood pressure.

Liberating yourself from the need to take prescription medications is a significant accomplishment—congratulations if you've been able to make this change in your life. If you're still relying on medications to reduce risk and minimize symptoms, that's okay—if you continue to follow our eating plan and exercise guidelines, you may also minimize

DINNER:	CALORIES	FAT (G)
WOMEN: 4 ounces very lean/lean protein	140–220	0–12
OR: 3 ounces very lean/lean protein + 1 ounce cheese		
MEN: 6 ounces very lean/lean protein	210–330	0–18
OR: 5 ounces very lean/lean protein + 1 ounce cheese		
1 serving healthy fat (for very lean protein only)	45	5
3 or more servings nonstarchy vegetables	45	0
Choose one of the carbohydrate choices listed below:	60–100	0–3
1 cup berries or ½ cup fruit		
½ cup nonfat or low-fat flavored yogurt		
1 cup nonfat or low-fat milk		
½ cup cooked beans		

SNACK

WOMEN: 1 per day between lunch and dinner
MEN: 2 per day, 1 between breakfast and lunch, and 1 between lunch and dinner

Select one of these options per snack:	CALORIES	FAT (G)
2 hardboiled eggs (yolk removed) + 4 tbsp. hummus (fill egg whites with hummus)	135	4–6
2 ounces very lean protein + 1 cup berries	130	0–2
20/20 High Protein Dry Powder Breakfast Shake served with 1 cup berries (no nut butter)	260	0
20/20 High Protein Ready to Drink Breakfast Shake served with 1 cup berries (no nut butter)	220	6

or eliminate the cost, inconvenience, and potential side effects of prescription medications.

For Stage 6, exercise will be as follows:

Level 1, Low Fitness: High-speed walking 5 minutes, running or hill walking 10 minutes; repeat three consecutive times for a total of 45 minutes of exercise. Complete at least 5 days per week. Maintain a pace that allows you to stay within your optimum heart rate (between 65 percent and 85 percent of your maximum).

Level 2, Moderate Fitness: High-speed walking 10 minutes, running or hill walking 30 minutes, high-speed walking 5 minutes. Complete at least 5 days per week. Maintain a pace that allows you to stay within your optimum heart rate (between 65 percent and 85 percent of your maximum).

Level 3, High Fitness: Running 6 miles, 4 days per week (fifth day is optional), plus running 8 miles, 1 day per week. Continue running gradual hills and keeping your heart rate at your optimum level. Has your pace improved? If so, keep pushing yourself and pursue a new goal, working toward completing 6 miles in 48 minutes or better.

All Levels: Continue to aim for 6,000 or more steps taken per day, outside of any exercise you're completing. Track your step progress with your pedometer.

Stage 6 Lifestyle Plan: Mindful Eating

It's time to check in on your eating habits. Removing mindless eating habits is important to creating long-term weight loss success, which is why we hope you've made an effort to practice mindful eating instead (see page 90). Mindful eating means that you focus on the act of eating instead of on the TV, computer, or smartphone. When these distractions are in place, it's all too easy to consume excess calories without even realizing it. Remember these important tips to help ensure you're mindful of what you're putting in your body:

- **Savor and enjoy the flavors of your food!** Pause before you begin eating to be thankful for the meal in front of you.
- **Minimize distractions while eating:** Sit down at the dinner table to enjoy your food; keep the TV off and put your smartphone and computer in the other room.
- **Consume food slowly:** Give yourself time to chew, taste, and swallow. This will allow your body a bit of time to process what you've eaten, increasing satiety and decreasing the chances of overeating.

CHAPTER 12

Stage 7: Grains and Starchy Vegetables

Welcome to the seventh stage of the Love Diet! You have likely experienced incredible results so far, and you should be proud of the efforts you've made to improve your health. By the time you've reached this stage, the changes you've made to your diet and exercise habits and to your overall mindset should have produced impressive and noticeable results: significant weight loss, a trimmer waist, increased energy, a calmer and clearer mind, reduced stress, and more. And with this stage, we will continue along the same path—there's no looking back!

In this final stage of the eating plan, you will be introducing whole grains back into your diet. This includes whole grain bread, rice, pasta, and cereal, and even snack foods such as pretzels and crackers. Starchy vegetables, such as corn, peas, potatoes, sweet potatoes, and winter squash, will also be reintroduced. While these foods are not whole grains, they have a similar carbohydrate and caloric content to grains and therefore can be categorized as such.

We advise caution when it comes to reintroducing whole grains into your diet. While they are better for you than refined grains—foods like white bread, white rice, white pasta, and anything made with white flour—they are still carbohydrates, which means they can leave you feeling hungry and can lead to overeating.

Guidelines for Eating Grains

We have seen grains create problems for many individuals in our program. In some cases, it's about the return of eating patterns and habits built up around grain-based carbohydrates. Most problem foods are a type of grain food. If you used to over-snack on chips and crackers or couldn't stop at just one roll with dinner, you will want to pay careful attention when you start eating the whole grain varieties of these foods. Here are some guidelines we've established to help ensure that you can enjoy grains without sabotaging your weight loss success:

Eat the right number of servings: During Stage 7, you can eat one 60- to 100-calorie whole grain serving per day. One slice of whole grain bread is typically around 100 calories. This means you can eat half a sandwich at a meal, but not a whole sandwich—the latter would be two servings of grains.

For other whole grains, such as brown rice, wild rice, and quinoa, you will measure your serving from the cooked grain. A ½ cup of each of these foods will provide you with about 100 calories.

As for starchy vegetables, the quantity that you can eat for 100 calories or less varies based on the vegetable. For corn and peas, it is ½ cup; for potatoes, it's one small potato, about 4 ounces. Because there's so much variation, it's recommended that you check calorie counts and serving sizes for other starchy vegetables that you add to your diet. (See also the Nutrition Summary on page 168 for additional starchy vegetable serving sizes.)

Ease them back into your diet: We recommend that for the first week you add one serving every other day. This will help prevent cravings and weight gain and allow you to develop a certain level of confidence with grains. Once you feel comfortable, and as long as you're not experiencing hunger cravings, bloating, or distress, you can increase it to one serving every day. Remember, your grain serving in that meal is your only carbohydrate source for that meal.

Don't introduce grains at snack times: The problem with most grain-based snack foods is that they're not high enough in protein to satiate. You will also find that 100 calories of snack foods is not much, leaving you in the precarious state of hungry and in the presence of problem foods. Even something that sounds like a balanced snack—cheese and crackers—is risky. Depending on the size and type of crackers, you might be able to have anywhere from four to ten crackers, which is enough to trigger your reward center and turn on your appetite, ultimately prompting you to reach for more.

Avoid grains when dining out: Bread served at restaurants is rarely whole grain and tends to be calorie dense. Plus, when there's a whole basket in front of you, stopping at one slice can be difficult. For items like rice or potatoes, restaurants will often serve significantly more than the ½ cup or so serving that is recommended. You don't need a heaping serving of pasta salad or a baked potato the size of a small football, especially when you can order a more satisfying plate filled with protein and vegetables.

Remember, grains aren't a required part of your daily nutrition: Even though previous dietary recommendations may have taught you otherwise, you don't need grains to function at your best. This is especially important for you if you have discovered that your body or weight loss is sensitive to them. Your body and brain need carbohydrates, but you can get sufficient amounts from berries, fruits, dairy, legumes, and vegetables. If introducing grains makes you hungry or tired, or gives you digestive problems, take them back out of your meal plan permanently. Plenty of participants in the 20/20 LifeStyles program have limited or avoided grains, and they've been very successful in both weight loss and weight maintenance.

Skip the grains that give you trouble: You might notice that some grains, but not all, create issues for you. Whole grain bread might be a trigger food for you, but you can eat whole wheat pasta without feeling the return of carb cravings or excess hunger. In this case, you would be wise to omit whole grain bread from your diet or only eat it on special occasions. If you notice that a certain whole grain food creates appetite issues for you, pay special attention to what you're pairing it with. For example, cereal and milk is a pairing of two carbohydrates, which makes it unlikely that this combo will keep you full; in fact, it might just make you hungrier. Instead of cereal and milk, try topping a serving of Greek yogurt with a little bit of cereal—this way you'll get some protein as well, which will better satisfy your appetite.

The Slim Plate

In Stage 7, we're going to introduce a new concept called the Slim Plate. The Slim Plate is a very basic tool that will help teach you how to plan meals by providing a visual of what your plate should look like. Understanding the makeup of this plate will be especially useful as you move toward your long-term, maintenance way of eating.

With the Slim Plate, one third of your plate should be protein, one third should be your nonstarchy vegetable servings, and the last third should be your one carbohydrate choice. When you eat according to this plate model, you are ensuring that you get a balanced amount of protein, vegetables, and carbohydrates. Here is what the plate looks like (you'll learn more about the plate model in the maintenance chapter):

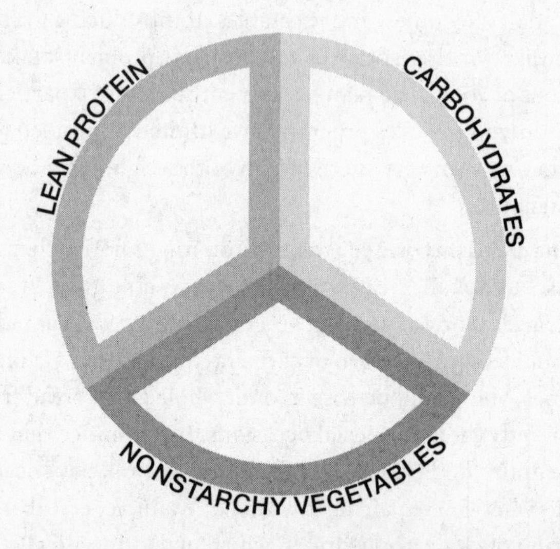

One tip to keep your portions balanced is to make sure you're using plates that are nine inches in diameter. Many plates have grown in size and can be as big as fourteen inches in diameter. A larger plate size can tempt you to fill the plate with bigger servings than you need. Smaller plates, on the other hand, can accommodate just as much food as you need and will appear fuller. This visual trick will help increase appetite satisfaction and make sticking to your serving sizes easier.

The Whole Grain Story: Options and Serving Sizes

All of the foods that can be added to your meals this stage are carbohydrates that you can enjoy with breakfast, lunch, or dinner. But remember, only one serving from the whole grain category is recommended per day, preferably with a meal and not as a snack.

Your whole grain options this stage are: whole grain breads, cooked whole grains, and whole grain cereals and crackers. The serving sizes will vary based on the food you choose but should always fall within the 60- to 100-calorie range.

Here are specific guidelines, serving sizes, and buying recommendations for the various types of whole grains you can enjoy during this stage (if a food label is provided, please refer to the nutrition label for more accurate nutrition facts).

Whole Grain Breads and Tortillas

Look for bread and tortilla varieties with the word *whole* and without the word *enriched* listed as part of the first ingredient. They should also contain:

- 3 grams or more of fiber per serving
- 3 grams or less of sugar per serving
- approximately 100 calories per serving with 15 to 20 grams of carbohydrates

SHOPPING FOR WHOLE GRAINS

It's not always easy to determine which breads and cereals are truly whole grain, especially when you're dealing with misleading labels. Follow these tips to help ensure you buy only the healthiest whole grains:

Look for the word *whole* first in the ingredients: The first grain listed, and every grain thereafter, should be identified as whole. Skip foods with refined grains.

Don't be fooled by healthy-sounding terms: Terms such as *100% wheat*, *multigrain*, and *cracked wheat* have nothing to do with whether the bread or cereal is whole grain or not.

Look for *100% whole grain* or *whole wheat* on the ingredient label: This ensures that you will get whole grains and not refined ones, which have been stripped of fiber and nutrients.

Know that the color of a food means nothing about its nutritional value: Just because a bread is brown or dark brown doesn't mean it's healthy—these darker hues can easily be added to foods with molasses or food coloring.

Buy for fiber too: Choose whole grain breads with at least 2 grams of fiber per slice and whole grain cereals with at least 8 grams of fiber per serving. You'll find the fiber count in the ingredients box on the label.

One serving is one slice or 100 calories. The following brands meet these guidelines:

- Oroweat 100% Whole Wheat Bread
- Oroweat Sandwich Thins
- Ezekiel 4:9 Bread (all varieties)
- Franz 100% Whole Wheat Bread
- Dave's Killer Bread (Thin-Sliced)
- Flatout Bread
- La Tortilla Factory whole wheat tortillas
- Mission Carb Balance whole wheat tortillas
- Thomas' Light Multi-Grain English Muffins

Cooked Whole Grains

One serving is ½ cup cooked or 100 calories.

- Bulgur
- Rice varieties: wild,* brown, forbidden black rice, brown basmati
- Whole wheat couscous
- Quinoa
- Steel cut oats
- Barley millet
- Amaranth
- Whole wheat pasta
- Brown rice pasta

Quick-and-Easy Whole Grain Meals

- ½ cup whole wheat couscous with 4 ounces shrimp and 1½ cups asparagus
- ½ cup whole wheat pasta with 4 ounces chicken sausage or turkey meatballs combined with ½ cup chopped bell pepper, ½ cup onions, and ½ cup tomatoes
- ½ cup quinoa with 1½ cups stir-fried mixed vegetables and chopped chicken

Whole Grain Snacks and Cereals

For cereals and whole grain snacks, the limit per serving is 100 calories, and the serving size will vary.

SNACKS

- Ak-mak crackers
- TLC crackers
- Wasa crackers

---

* Be wary of wild rice blends; they can contain non–whole grain rice varieties.

- Mary's Gone Crackers
- Whole wheat matzos
- Snyder's whole wheat pretzels
- 100-calorie bags of popcorn
- Newman's Own, Light Popcorn
- Van's Multi-Grain Toaster Waffles

COLD CEREALS

For cold cereals, be sure to choose varieties that have less than 9 grams of sugar and at least 3 grams of fiber per serving, like these varieties:

- Kellogg's All-Bran
- Barbara's Shredded Spoonfuls
- Barbara's Honest O's
- Barbara's Puffins Multigrain
- Kashi GoLean cereals
- Kashi Good Friends Original Cereal
- Nature's Path Flax Plus
- General Mills Multi Grain Cheerios
- Post Grape-Nuts
- Post Shredded Wheat

HOT CEREALS

The serving size for hot cereals is ½ cup cooked. Try these brands:

- Arrowhead Mills
- Bob's Red Mill
- Hodgson Mill
- Nature's Path
- Quaker Oats (rolled or steel cut)

The Other Whole Grain: Starchy Vegetables

With starchy vegetables, it's important to be very mindful of servings, as many of these foods can lead to overeating if not measured carefully. One serving of starchy vegetables is 60 to 100 calories, approximately 15 to 20 grams of carbohydrates. Again, starchy vegetables count as a carbohydrate food choice. Specific servings are as follows:

Corn: 1 serving = ½ cup

Peas: 1 serving = ½ cup

Potatoes, yams, sweet potatoes: 1 serving = 1 small 4-ounce potato cooked or ½ cup mashed

Acorn, butternut, pumpkin, and other winter squash: 1 serving = ½ cup cubed

Preparing Starchy Vegetables

In restaurants or in traditional home cooking, starchy vegetables are often fried or prepared with butter, sugar, maple syrup, sour cream, cheese, and other high-calorie toppings. However, there are healthy and tasty alternative ways to prepare starchy vegetables. Here are some of our favorite methods for cooking or prepping starchy vegetables:

- Use low-sodium chicken broth instead of butter on mashed potatoes.
- Add cinnamon, nutmeg, and a splash of orange juice to ½ cup pureed winter squash. Top with walnut or pecan halves and bake for a side dish of carbohydrates plus healthy fat.
- Bake a small potato or sweet potato spears (serving size 4 ounces) on a baking sheet coated with cooking spray at 400°F for 30 to 35 minutes. For even more flavor, sprinkle with herbs or spices such as paprika, pumpkin pie spice, chili seasoning, or garlic powder before baking.

STAGE 7 NUTRITION SPECIFICS

Women: 1,100–1,400 calories per day
Men: 1,300–1,700 calories per day

BREAKFAST:	CALORIES	FAT (G)
4 ounces very lean protein	140	0–4
2 servings healthy fat (page 101)	90	10
Choose one of the carbohydrate choices listed below:		
½ cup fruit or 1 cup berries	60–80	0
1 serving whole grains or starchy vegetable	100	0
OR: 20/20 High Protein Dry Powder Breakfast Shake made with 1 cup berries and 1 tablespoon nut butter	360	10
OR: 20/20 High Protein Ready to Drink Breakfast Shake served with 1 cup berries and 1 tablespoon nut butter	309	14

LUNCH:	CALORIES	FAT (G)
WOMEN: 4 ounces very lean/lean protein	140–220	0–12
OR: 3 ounces very lean/lean protein + 1 ounce cheese		
MEN: 6 ounces very lean/lean protein	210–330	0–18
OR: 5 ounces very lean/lean protein + 1 ounce cheese		
1 serving healthy fat (for very lean protein only)	45	5
3 or more servings nonstarchy vegetables	45	0
Choose one of the carbohydrate choices listed below:	60–100	0–3
1 cup berries		
½ cup fruit		
½ cup nonfat or low-fat flavored yogurt		
1 cup nonfat or low-fat milk		
½ cup cooked beans		
1 serving whole grains or starchy vegetable*		

- Top a small baked potato with nonfat plain or Greek yogurt, salsa, or low-fat cheese instead of sour cream or butter.
- Sprinkle corn or peas on a mixed green salad.

Stage 7 Nutrition Summary

This stage sees the addition of whole grains to your meals. This includes whole grain breads, cooked whole grains, whole grain cereals and crackers, and starchy vegetables. Eat only one serving per day from this category, with specific servings as follows:

DINNER:	CALORIES	FAT (G)
WOMEN: 4 ounces very lean/lean protein	140–220	0–12
OR: 3 ounces very lean/lean protein + 1 ounce cheese		
MEN: 6 ounces very lean/lean protein	210–330	0–18
OR: 5 ounces very lean/lean protein + 1 ounce cheese		
1 serving healthy fat (for very lean protein only)	45	5
3 or more servings nonstarchy vegetables	45	0
Choose one of the carbohydrate choices listed below:	60–100	0–3
1 cup berries		
½ cup fruit		
½ cup nonfat or low-fat flavored yogurt		
1 cup nonfat or low-fat milk		
1 serving whole grain or starchy vegetable*		
½ cup cooked beans		

SNACK

WOMEN: 1 per day between lunch and dinner

MEN: 2 per day, 1 between breakfast and lunch, and 1 between lunch and dinner

Select one of these options per snack:	CALORIES	FAT (G)
2 light string cheese sticks + ½ cup fruit	180	5
¼ cup hummus + ½ cup mixed vegetables	130	4–6
2 ounces very lean protein + 1 cup berries	130	0–2
20/20 High Protein Dry Powder Breakfast Shake made with 1 cup berries (no nut butter)	260	0
20/20 High Protein Ready to Drink Breakfast Shake served with 1 cup berries (no nut butter)	220	6

* Consume only one whole grain or starchy vegetable serving per day.

- Whole grain bread: 1 serving = 1 slice or 100 calories
- Cooked whole grains: 1 serving = ½ cup cooked or 100 calories
- Cereals and whole grain snacks: 1 serving = 100 calories
- Starchy vegetables: 1 serving = 60–100 calories

    Corn: 1 serving = ½ cup

    Peas: 1 serving = ½ cup

    Potatoes, yams, sweet potatoes: 1 serving = 1 small 4-ounce potato cooked, or ½ cup mashed

- Acorn, butternut, pumpkin, and other winter squash: 1 serving = ½ cup cubed

Stage 7 Exercise Plan: I Am Amazing

You're now in great shape. For many of you, this will be the best physical condition of your adult life so far. The best part about this is that your fitness will only continue to improve as you keep gifting your body with exercise. Now's the time to reach out and try something you've dreamed about, something from your own personal bucket list. Have you ever wanted to run a marathon, do a triathlon, climb a mountain, go on a bicycle tour, or join an adult sports league? Start planning to make it happen. Begin by seeking out training guides online or hiring a coach in the specific area in which you'd like to excel. And don't be shy about your next quest—ask friends and family if they've ever tried the specific activity or event you're considering. Most people are eager to share their experience and offer insider advice.

For Stage 7, exercise will be as follows:

Level 1, Low Fitness: Running or hill walking 15 minutes, high-speed walking 10 minutes; repeat two consecutive times for a total of 50 minutes. Complete this workout at least 5 days per week. Maintain a pace that allows you to stay within your optimum heart rate (between 65 percent and 85 percent of your maximum).

Level 2, Moderate Fitness: Running or hill walking 40 minutes, high-speed walking 10 minutes. Complete this workout at least 5 days per week. Maintain a pace that allows you to stay within your optimum heart rate (between 65 percent and 85 percent of your maximum).

Level 3, High Fitness: Running 6 miles 4 days per week and 8 miles 1 day per week. Optional sixth workout of the week: 6 miles. Continue running gradual hills and monitoring your pace. Maintain a pace that allows you to keep your heart rate at your optimum level. Your goal is now to complete 6 miles in 45 minutes or better.

All Levels: Keep wearing your pedometer when not exercising, aiming to reach 6,000 steps per day, excluding your workouts.

Stage 7 Lifestyle Plan: Reasonable Expectations

We know that this is the last time you want to have to lose a substantial amount of weight, but have you made this point clear to yourself? As you work toward completing the seventh stage of the Love Diet and moving into a maintenance plan, it's important to reflect on the work you've done. Pause to consider all the incredible effort you've made; the self-defeating habits (eating and emotional) you've given up; and the productive, healing, and health-restoring ones you've gained. Just marvel for a moment about how far you've come. It feels good, doesn't it? Being able to see and celebrate the new you—the dynamic and energetic individual who you knew was there all along.

As you look toward living your life outside of a structured plan, it's also important that you begin to steel yourself against the many forces that can threaten your success. The environmental issues that contributed to your weight gain are likely still there, whether they involve being subjected to the constant marketing of unhealthful food and drink or being targeted by the diet assassins in your life. Difficulties will present themselves, and there will be times when they push you off track. You might lose control of your time or be talked into skipping exercise or eating foods off your plan, and you might gain back some of the weight as a consequence.

But here's what you won't do: you won't let yourself continue sliding the wrong way, all the way back into your old habits. You won't let yourself because you know better now—you know now that health is a gift to yourself, a reflection of the love you have for yourself and something you're not willing to give up.

In the next chapter, we'll explore maintenance further and introduce techniques to help you stay committed to the eating and exercise principles you've learned. As you complete this final stage of the plan, begin to visualize yourself transitioning into a maintenance phase, free from the structured stages, but still eating and exercising to create the best you. See yourself healthy, happy, and confident with the commitment you've made to put your health first.

CHAPTER 13

Welcome to Your Future: Maintaining Your Weight Loss and Your New Health

Congratulations on reaching the maintenance stage of the Love Diet! Be sure to take the time to commend yourself on this accomplishment—you were able to find and focus the self-love and dedication needed to create a profound life change—that's something to be incredibly proud of.

Your commitment and efforts have paid off: you look and feel wonderful; your friends, family, and coworkers are amazed at your success; you have begun to buy clothes that you never thought would look good on you; and you are engaging in physical activities at a level you didn't think was possible. Being this new you is an invigorating and powerful experience, and because of all the positive changes you've made, you feel energized and confident about who you are and how you live your life.

The question is: how do you make these feelings last forever? Or maybe you're asking, "How do I sustain the results I've worked so hard for?" or "How do I keep from falling back into my old habits?" These are critical questions to answer because as challenging as losing weight and getting into great physical shape might have been for you, that was actually the easier part of your journey to lifelong health. The hardest part is continuing on the same path so that you maintain, and even improve, your health and weight loss. (If you have ever dieted successfully and then struggled to maintain your results, you know this truth all too well.)

Part of the difficulty in maintaining healthy habits is that the food environment remains as challenging as ever. Fast-food restaurants are still everywhere selling cheap, convenient food, and processed, refined carbs still taunt you from nearly every aisle in the grocery store—or these days, from nearly every aisle in *every* store. (Those shelves filled with junk food by the cashier at bookstores, sporting goods stores, and clothing stores? They're called impulse aisles for a reason—don't give in!) But the good news is that *you* have changed. You have gained a new level of nutrition knowledge and have developed a fierce commitment to caring for yourself as you care for those you love—these are powerful forces against a deleterious environment.

The key to creating lasting success is harnessing yourself to the positive motivation that has gotten you this far. Maintaining motivation isn't about being overly strict or hard on yourself but instead about giving yourself the time to make progress to the point where your healthy new lifestyle becomes permanent. Even though you've likely spent several weeks following the Seven Stages, your healthy habits are still in relative infancy—if you give them time and patience, they will grow and mature into unshakeable, fully formed skills that make staying on track simple.

There are techniques and steps you can take to help make sure you are successful in maintaining the results from the Seven Stages. Here are some of the proven strategies for creating continued success:

1. Be aware of lapses—and respond to them with love, not criticism. One of the most important factors in maintaining motivation is staying tethered to your newfound self-love and self-acceptance. This means maintaining a positive attitude and allowing yourself to have slipups without resorting to negative self-talk or self-condemnation. Specifically, it means making room for lapses but ensuring that you stop short of a relapse into your old lifestyle. A lapse is when you allow your eating or exercise habits to fall off track once; a relapse is a prolonged episode of bad habits. Lapses will happen, because you are human and you cannot maintain perfection indefinitely. The key is to recognize a lapse early on and take action, thereby preventing a relapse (we'll introduce a relapse prevention plan later in the chapter).

If you lapse and eat an unhealthful food or slack on exercise, you should acknowledge responsibility but should not fall into the shame cycle (more on the shame cycle on page 15) or get stuck in a bubble of blame. Acknowledge a slipup by saying, "Yes, I did that," and then get right back on track. Reject the negative thoughts in your head that try to tell you you're a failure, a bad person, or a weak person or that you're out of control (revisit the section on positive self-talk on page 47). From there, you can take the time to analyze what went wrong—why did you fall off track? What can help you stick to your plan in the future? Use any lapses as learning experiences to help strengthen your commitment skills.

2. *Establish yellow- and red-light points for your weight.* If you begin to lose control of your healthy eating habits, it's usually not immediately noticeable. The scale will reveal a delayed truth, often only showing movement after a few days. This is why it's recommended that you continue to use your tracker for up to two years after you've reached your weight loss goal—maintaining an awareness of what you're eating will help prevent a slide into disordered eating.

You can also create warning weight points to help slow or stop a slide in the wrong direction. We call these points your yellow-light and red-light weights. Your yellow-light weight should be three pounds above your maintenance weight, and your red-light point should be five pounds above your maintenance weight.

If you reach your yellow-light point, you must take corrective action by getting reconnected with your commitment to give yourself the gift of health. If you reach your red-light point, you need to reconnect with a support person or group—a friend, family member, or even online forum that will come to your aid with encouragement to get back on track. You can also go back to Stage 2 for a week or more—this stage is your safe place that will always work to get you back into balance. It's essential that you act quickly before any of your old bad habits begin to settle in and get comfortable.

3. *Renew your contract with yourself.* Remember the contract you wrote with yourself before you began the Seven Stages? Now would be a good time to revisit that contract and renew it. Just like couples who renew their vows, you can go back to freshen up on the commitment

you've made to yourself. This exercise can rejuvenate your motivation and remind you of the healthy habits you've adopted and why it's so important to stick to them. Remember, you deserve to be happy and healthy, and to treat yourself with love. You've worked very hard to get to this point and you deserve to keep the weight off, have increased energy, and enjoy an improved quality of life.

When you renew your contract, be specific and don't be afraid to get creative. Don't just write, *I promise to eat healthfully and go to the gym at least four to five times a week*. Instead, think about a goal you're excited to pursue—a door that your new health has opened for you. Maybe you want to improve your walking or running pace and eventually work up to entering a local race. Or maybe you want to complete a nearby hike. Or perhaps you want to learn three new dishes you can cook for your family. Write down your goal and what it might take for you to get there. For example, you could write: *I will continue to exercise five times a week and improve my pace to a ten-minute mile.* Or, *I will take a healthy cooking class so I can learn how to make new meals for myself and my family.* Pick something that's challenging enough to keep you motivated and then start working toward it—this is what Kurt did before he found himself on the peak of Mount Rainier in Washington State a few years after first visiting us at 20/20 LifeStyles.

When Kurt first came to us, he had fully accepted who he was physically. He exercised occasionally and played golf once in a while, but his fitness was severely limited by his weight and he figured it always would be because he didn't really know how to change. Then, at age forty, Kurt was diagnosed with type 2 diabetes, high blood pressure, high triglycerides, and high cholesterol—and he was 310 pounds, obese for his six-foot frame. Change was no longer optional; it was critical.

His doctor laid out a plan: Kurt would go on medication immediately and would likely need to stay on it forever. And even with pharmaceutical intervention, he faced a potentially shortened lifespan. Kurt was stunned. He knew his health hadn't been perfect for quite some time, but this was beyond what he was prepared to hear.

He began to do some research, wondering what a life filled with prescription medication would look and feel like. He read about statins, blood pressure meds, and insulin injections, should it ever come to that. And he read about the side effects associated with all of these medications, thinking about which ones he might have to endure. Suddenly, Kurt made a promise to himself—he wasn't going to go on medications; he would find another way.

A friend steered him toward our clinic, which seemed like a good fit given our emphasis on treating metabolic disorders. The complete lifestyle program he was introduced to (the very same one you've followed in this book) seemed promising—it would give him the education he needed on how to live a healthy lifestyle. Looking back, Kurt says deciding to follow the program likely saved his life.

Kurt never had to take a single drug. He lost 110 pounds and reversed his metabolic disorders—he got rid of his type 2 diabetes, high cholesterol, and high blood pressure, and he gained energy, endurance, and an impressive level of fitness. Kurt truly feels as though he beat the system.

During the maintenance stage, he began to really get into hiking and mountain climbing. He set big goals to hike high peaks, and he worked hard to build his fitness so he could meet these goals—and he did. Kurt hiked fourteen-thousand-foot Mount Rainier three times. He also successfully hiked mountains in South America and Gannett Peak in Wyoming.

Looking back, Kurt remembers how he used to have trouble climbing a flight of stairs—and now he's successfully climbing mountains; he never would have imagined his life could have changed as much as it did. Kurt's transformation started the day he decided to take his health into his own hands, and it continued when he challenged himself beyond the Seven Stages and pushed himself to keep pursuing new goals.

Kurt's story shows us that the maintenance stage can be about so much more than just maintaining—it can present the chance to truly explore your new abilities and redefine your potential.

4. *Continue to use visualization.* Visualization is a wonderful technique to help sustain motivation. Many athletes and people at the top of their professional game use visualization to help produce consistent success. The famous basketball player Michael Jordan would visualize his shots over and over before he attempted them. This way, he said, when it actually came time to shoot, he would feel as though he had already shot—and scored—many times before. You can achieve that

same success by seeing yourself maintain your healthy habits in several different scenarios. When you visualize yourself successfully performing health-affirming habits, like turning down the hors d'oeuvres tray, ordering sparkling water instead of alcohol, or putting on your running shoes and heading out the door for a workout, you will automatically follow through with these actions when the time comes to act them out in real life.

5. Weigh yourself daily, or at least weekly. Avoiding the scale is a sure sign of imminent relapse. If you find you have not weighed in for over a week, it's time to check in with your weight and make sure you've maintained. If you haven't and you've instead reached your yellow- or red-light point (see page 175), it's imperative that you get serious about getting back on track. Keep in mind that if you've noticed a return of cravings, you can always return to Stage 2 for a week or more to restore balance to your metabolism.

6. Beware of portion bloat. When you stop weighing and measuring your food, it's inevitable that your portions will start to expand. This is especially true with carbohydrates, which can easily grow beyond the recommended ½ cup or tennis ball–size portion. To avoid losing sight of proper portions, we recommend that you go back to weighing and measuring your food at least one week per month.

7. Stay in control of your time. Managing your time is crucial to maintaining success with your eating, sleep, and exercise habits. If you begin to lose control of time, it won't be long before your habits begin to shift and your stress levels start to increase. Once your stress levels increase, you will begin to produce more cortisol, which will trigger cravings and promote the storage of fat. Sticking to your commitment to carve out time for food preparation and exercise will prevent this whole cycle from gaining momentum.

8. Never skip workouts. There are so many convincing reasons for skipping workouts, which is why it's important that you get a workout buddy—being accountable to another person is one of the best ways to ensure you stick with your exercise goals. Hopefully, you were able to rely on a workout buddy throughout the Seven Stages and you can continue to do so. If you couldn't find someone at your fitness level at the time, perhaps your improved fitness will open the door to other individuals. Think about your neighbors, coworkers, or if you're a parent, maybe another parent at your kid's school—you never know who is looking for a reliable workout partner just like you. If you have difficulty finding a workout buddy, sign up for a class at your local health club or community center, which will give you a schedule that can help keep you accountable. Or consider joining a recreational sports team—this way you'll have a whole team depending upon you to show up and break a sweat!

9. Continue to grow your nutrition knowledge. After reading this book, you will have gained an impressive amount of knowledge about health and nutrition, knowledge that can be considered the roots of your new lifestyle. If you continue to feed and nourish your new lifestyle with even more information, it will only grow stronger and more secure, helping you branch out further away from your old habits. You can check out some of the many resources available to you on our website at 2020lifestyles.com, and if you have the 20/20 LifeStyles app, be sure to check out the Resources and Tools section where you will find knowledge-building information.

10. Eat the Love Diet way for life. Once you've achieved your goal weight by following the Seven Stages, you can transition to what we call the maintenance meal plan. Since you've already added the various food groups back into your diet, the goal now is to eat a balanced diet that allows you to successfully maintain your new weight for the rest of your life.

The biggest change as you transition to the maintenance phase is your total caloric intake. Once you reach your goal weight, you will need to slowly increase your calories so that you stop losing weight and instead start maintaining it. Let's review how to determine the specific maintenance calorie intake for your body and how you will modify the Slim Plate moving forward.

Determining Your Maintenance Calorie Range

Figuring out your personal maintenance calorie range is the most customized way to make sure your body gets just what it needs to maintain your weight loss. That's because it depends upon your distinct profile, specifically your age, gender, height, weight, and activity level.

To determine your maintenance calorie range, you have to first determine your basal metabolic rate (BMR), which is the amount of calories your body burns at rest. You can find several BMR calculators on websites like www.bmrcalculator.org.

Once you have your BMR, you will multiply this number by your activity level. If you have a moderate activity level, you will multiply your BMR by 1.2; and for a high activity level, you will multiply your BMR by 1.4.

Let's look at an example with a thirty-nine-year-old woman named Brenda who is five foot seven and 130 pounds with a high activity level. Brenda works in a restaurant and is walking and carrying dishes eight hours a day. She also works out vigorously four days per week. When she plugs her height and weight into a BMR calculator, she learns that her BMR is 1,300 calories per day without any extra activity. Now, given her high activity level, Brenda will multiply 1,300 by 1.4 and get 1,820. This is her approximate maintenance daily calorie intake.

But Brenda won't make an immediate jump to eating 1,820 calories per day after she's completed the Seven Stages. Instead, she will look back at what she was eating when she completed Stage 7 and gradually increase her calorie intake by 100 calories per week until she reaches her personalized maintenance intake. If she was eating 1,400 calories when she reached her goal weight, she will eat 1,500 during the second week of maintenance, 1,600 during the third, and so on, until she reaches 1,820.

When you've determined your own BMR, be sure to multiply this figure by your activity level. The resulting figure is your caloric goal for the maintenance phase, which you will get to, as Brenda did, by increasing your intake by 100 calories each week. The easiest ways to add 100 calories to your daily intake are to enjoy a 100-calorie snack during the day or to add extra protein or a healthy fat serving to a meal, such as a ¼ avocado or 12 almonds.

To increase your calories properly—so as to avoid weight gain—you will need to use both your tracker and your scale. Your tracker will allow you to document your calories consumed each day and will provide a reliable record of where you should be with your calories each week, and the scale will help you pinpoint the caloric intake that keeps your weight constant. Consider this a little bit of diet detective work to make sure you're eating the right amount for your body and for your ideal weight.

Here's how you will use the scale: Weigh yourself the day before you increase your intake by 100 calories. Then, after one week of eating at your new level of calories, weigh yourself again. If your weight decreased, increase your intake by another 100 daily calories for the following week and continue until your weight remains constant or you reach your personalized maintenance intake.

When it comes to weight loss maintenance, meal tracking and healthy eating habits are the most important pieces of success. Some people think that they can return to their poor dietary habits and still maintain their weight loss because they're exercising—and this may be true for a short period of time, but ultimately you can't out-exercise a bad diet. All of the individuals in the 20/20 LifeStyles program who relied on large amounts of exercise to balance out a poor diet eventually gained their weight back—don't make the same mistake! Injuries, illness, time conflicts, and so on will inevitably get in the way of exercise at times, but you can always make healthy food choices.

Modifying the Slim Plate for Maintenance

In Stage 7, we introduced the Slim Plate to you as a way to help you visualize the macronutrient breakdown of your meals. In the maintenance stage, you will continue to compartmentalize your plate in a similar fashion. The nutritional stars will still be protein and vegetables because the goal remains to keep your body in metabolic balance, and these foods are the best for keeping you full and satisfied without promoting fat storage.

Breakfast Slim Plate

For breakfast, your plate will look very similar to the previous weeks. For men and women, whole food–based breakfasts should include 4 or more ounces of protein, two healthy fat servings, as many vegetable servings as you would like, and only one serving of carbohydrate. A few notes on breakfast during maintenance:

- Protein in the morning is crucial—if you're interested in maintaining your health and weight loss, having a protein-rich breakfast should undoubtedly become a lifelong habit.
- You may now want to include a grain-based food with your breakfast, such as a slice of whole wheat toast or steel cut oats.
- We have included vegetables on the breakfast plate because they're a wonderful way to add volume and fiber without adding a significant number of calories. Try adding spinach or kale to a morning protein shake, or bell peppers and onions to an omelet or scramble.
- If you want to add calories to your breakfast, increase your protein by 1 to 2 ounces and be sure to include two healthy fat servings.

Here's how your maintenance breakfast plate will look:

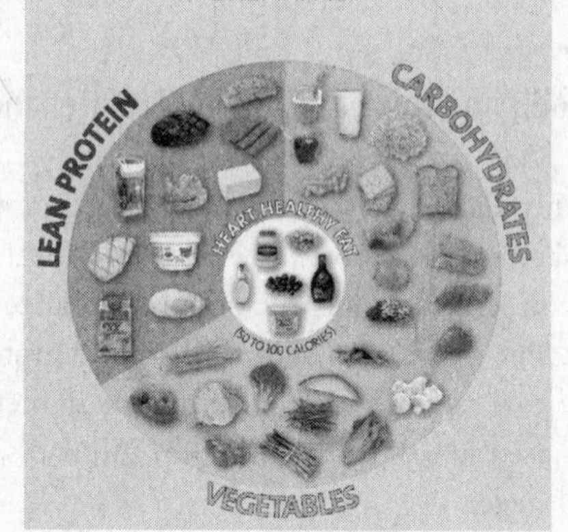

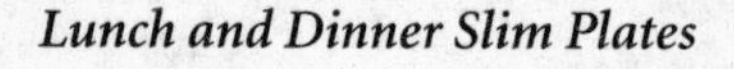

Lunch and Dinner Slim Plates

Your lunch and dinner plates should be approximately one third protein, one third carbohydrates, and one third vegetables, which is identical to the weight loss portion of the eating plan. Women should aim to eat 4 to 6 ounces of protein with lunch and dinner, while men should aim for a minimum of 6 to 8 ounces. Both men and women should include two healthy fat servings at lunch and dinner to bump up the calories in each meal.

If you find that you still need to increase your calories, it is best to add only lean protein or healthy fats. We strongly advise against using carbohydrates to increase your caloric intake. Just because your body has changed over the course of the Seven Stages doesn't mean carbohydrates have—when eaten in excess, they may trigger hunger, cravings, and weight gain.

If you eat fatty meats like bacon, lamb, pork or beef ribs, or higher-fat steak cuts like a prime rib or a rib eye, remember that these will be higher in calories and saturated fat than very lean and lean meats. Since you're looking to increase your calories during this stage, more calories isn't necessarily a bad thing, but it's best to track these foods and omit any additional fat servings with your meal.

Here is how your lunch and dinner plate will look:

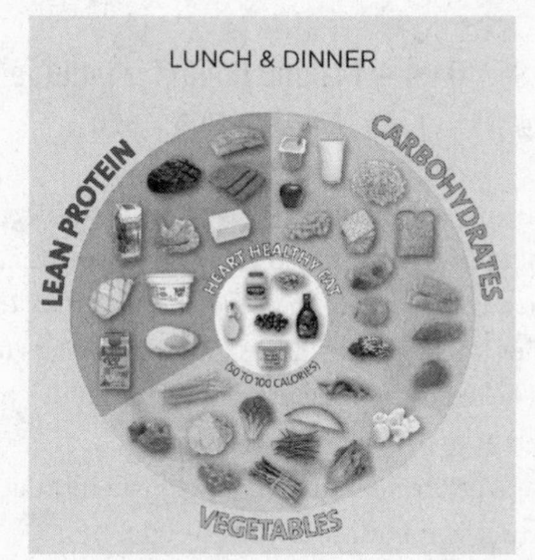

Where Do Snacks Fit on the Slim Plate?

While snacks don't fit on either of the main meal plate models during the maintenance stage, you can continue to eat snacks each day, increasing them to two or more to increase calorie intake as needed.

Select snacks that are smart and healthy pairings, approximately one serving of carbohydrate and one or two servings of healthy fat or lean protein. Examples of smart snacks include a small apple with approximately 1 tablespoon of nut butter, which adds about 200 calories to your daily intake, or 1 cup of carrots and 4 tablespoons of hummus, which will also provide about 200 calories. Smart snacks keep your energy levels up and your hunger satisfied.

A couple other notes on snacks:

- It's best to avoid eating grain-based foods alone as snacks, even during the maintenance stage. Foods such as crackers and cereals are too easy to overeat, and it's often difficult to include enough protein to offset the carbs.
- Unless you will be awake for over four hours after dinner, do not add a second snack after dinner. If you go to bed within four hours of dinner, dinner should be your last food for the day.

The 90/10 Rule: Making Room for Indulgences in the Maintenance Stage

Maintenance means being able to allow yourself indulgences from time to time, just not all of the time. To maintain your weight loss and the health you gained by following the Seven Stages, stick to the Slim Plate 90 percent of the time, using proteins and healthy fats to increase your daily calories. The other 10 percent of the time, allow yourself to enjoy something off plan, such as a glass of wine with dinner or a dessert. Use this 90/10 rule as a general guideline to help you indulge in moderation while ensuring that you maintain your weight.

Here are a few additional recommendations to keep in mind when indulging:

- Limit alcohol and desserts to portions that are less than 300 calories, and enjoy these treats no more than two times a week. With

DINING OUT FOR LIFE

When you dine out during maintenance, be sure to use the Slim Plate. In a restaurant, visualize your plate with the dividing lines that indicate one third protein, one third salad or vegetables, and the last third carbohydrates. If you order wine, limit yourself to one glass of wine and let this take the place of the carbohydrate in your meal. Beware of any grain-based side dishes since the portions will often be excessive and the grains used will rarely be whole grains. If you do order a grain side, you can make some modifications:

- Ask for a smaller amount than the typical serving.
- If you get the full serving, portion out ½ cup (eyeball it) and share the rest with a dining companion.
- Ask for a double portion of vegetables.
- Avoid any alcohol with your meal.

You may find that even with these adjustments, keeping your grain portions in check at restaurants is too difficult. If this is the case for you, skip them completely. Overeating carbohydrates can trigger shifts in your metabolic chemistry and bring back hunger and cravings, putting your new body and normal weight at risk.

alcohol, this means avoiding high-sugar beverages, such as daiquiris and margaritas, and choosing a 6-ounce glass of wine instead.

- When you enjoy indulgences, be sure to meal track, including documenting any noticeable increases in hunger. If you notice an increase in hunger, we recommend that you take that food or drink out of your diet again.
- Count any alcohol or dessert you consume as your carbohydrate for the meal. This means that if you have a glass of wine, you will omit the brown rice or other carbohydrate you would have otherwise had with a meal.

Keep in mind that these recommendations for the maintenance stage are made to help you solidify your new lifestyle to the point that it becomes second nature. You have worked so hard and love your new body, so make sure you remember this when you make your food choices. The pride you take in your appearance and your health should now filter into what you put into your body.

A Plan for Preventing a Lifestyle Relapse

At some point, you will feel incredibly confident about your commitment to your healthy new lifestyle—and while developing this level of confidence is the goal, it's also important to retain an awareness of how far you've come. If you lose track of your starting point entirely, you risk becoming overconfident, which can leave room for a sneaky slide back into your old lifestyle.

Over time, you might forget the pain of limited mobility, limited energy, clothes that don't fit, being out of breath from walking up the stairs, and having to take multiple medications for your metabolic disorders. And in the place of this pain, there might appear a sort of indulgence high, a false and fleeting joy you might feel after eating French fries, pastries, pancakes, or fresh bread. This can mark the slow and insidious beginning of a relapse.

You'll remember that a lapse is defined as a single event in which you lose self-control and then re-establish it. A relapse, on the other hand, is a significant, repeated loss of self-control—a series of lapses or slips—that can lead to you giving up. And once you've given up, it's only a matter of time until you regain your lost weight and your metabolic disorder comes back to life. (One way to help prevent this from occurring is to be sure to establish yellow-light and red-light weights; see page 175 for more on this.)

The goal is to manage lapses before they become relapses. Management isn't complicated, but it does involve being acutely aware of situations that may be challenging for you. We call these high-risk situations:

- A major increase in your stress due to work, family, or finances
- Having negative emotions like depression, anger, or fear
- Traveling

- Spending time with people who love to eat unhealthful foods
- Eating out
- Holidays
- Parties and celebrations
- A major change in your life, including marriage, divorce, having a child, moving, changing jobs
- A crisis with your parents or siblings
- Injury and illness

The first step in not letting these situations destroy all your hard work is to identify that the situation is there in the first place and then to take the time to center yourself as it relates to your eating and exercise habits. Remind yourself that following through with your commitments to yourself is the best thing you can do in any of these situations. Eating well and continuing to exercise will help you remain physically and mentally balanced, even in the face of some of the toughest life challenges.

If you do lapse, it's time to launch into the five-step relapse prevention protocol:

1. **Forgive yourself:** Go back to the self-acceptance, self-respect, and self-love you've developed for yourself and reconnect with these positive feelings. It's much easier to do good things for yourself when you love yourself.
2. **Analyze what you did wrong:** What did you do and why did you do it? Do not settle for the easy answers like "I just wanted to" or "I don't know." You may have to get out your journal or tablet to write until you find the real reason.
3. **Create a plan:** The Love Diet has given you all the tools you need for breaking destructive eating patterns, and the book will always be here for you. You can always begin again with the process, or return to Stage 2 to restore the foundation of your healthy eating habits.
4. **Visualize or rehearse your plan:** See yourself eating well and exercising again, and think about how good you'll feel to be back on track.

5. **Develop a plan for the next time:** Inevitably, you will find yourself in another high-risk situation—be ready for it by having a plan in place.

If reading about potential lapses and relapses makes you anxious, that's a good sign—a little fear about your future success is a good thing and will keep you motivated and vigilant.

How to Bring More Support Into Your Life

One technique that has helped many of our alumni maintain their weight loss is to start a maintainer group. You can reach out to friends, family, or coworkers—anyone you know who may want to work together to stay on track with healthy habits—to create a group. Explain that you want to put a friendly support group together to help keep yourself motivated and to help others stay motivated as well. You can share healthy recipes, reach out before a high-risk situation to get a bit of encouragement, and connect on any challenges you may still be having.

The group can become even more interactive when you arrange joint weigh-ins. In this case, you would need to meet at a central location on a certain day each week to weigh in. Each of you can share your yellow-light weight, and if your weight goes above that number, you have to put a dollar in the kitty. If you are still over the next week, the amount goes up to two dollars, and if you are not under your yellow-light weight by the third week and beyond, you have to contribute four dollars each week. Once a year, the group can collect the money and plan a fun event to do together. This is a very motivating and fun way to sustain accountability and support for maintaining your weight loss.

Another way to increase the support you receive on a daily basis—without needing anyone other than yourself—is to write positive affirmations and read them each day. Get out a stack of three-by-five cards and write a short affirmation on each card. Some examples are:

I accept, respect, and love myself.

I am feeling and thinking thin.

I love feeling healthy.

I am stronger today than yesterday.

I have more energy.

I've been eating and exercising right.

I'm a more productive and successful person.

I am improving in every way.

I'm learning more every day.

I'm looking good.

It's *so* worth it.

The best way to get back on plan is to not get off it.

I will follow my plan today.

I like the way my clothes fit and look.

I want to live to see my kids married.

Right after you get out of bed each morning, pick one card and read it. These messages will motivate and inspire you, helping to shape your attitude for the day.

Staying Connected to Love

As you make your way through the maintenance stage into permanent weight loss, it's vitally important to stay connected to the ultimate goal of the program: for you to learn to love yourself and to make choices for your health, body, and life that reflect this love. It is self-love and your new or renewed sense of self-acceptance and self-respect that will be the most critical factors in maintaining lifelong success.

If ever you find yourself slipping back into negative self-talk or you feel your commitments begin to weaken around any particular people or situations, step back and reconnect with the self-love you've worked so hard to develop. Think of it as a precious commodity that you refuse to surrender, even in the most challenging scenarios. When you stay love-centered, you won't even have to think about protecting your health—it will just come naturally to you, for the rest of your life.

PART IV

The Love Diet Seasonings, Recipes, and Meal Plans

CHAPTER 14

How to Spice Up the Love Diet: Seasonings, Marinades, and Rubs

The best part of eating healthfully on the Love Diet is discovering that you don't have to sacrifice flavor for your health. In fact, this chapter is going to make it even easier to stay slim and maintain your healthy new lifestyle with delicious marinades and rubs you can use throughout the Seven Stages. Think of this chapter as your go-to guide for quick and simple ways to boost flavor in some of your favorite meals. You'll also discover two flavorful cooking methods for adding more delicious options to your everyday meals throughout the Seven Stages: poaching and steaming. Both methods require little effort and time and will reward you with moist meats and fresh-tasting crisp veggies.

We hope you'll use many of the marinades, rubs, and poaching broths featured in this chapter. All of them are acceptable for use throughout the Seven Stages, from Stage 1 through Stage 7 and into maintenance. Because they all have less than 50 calories, you will not need to count the nutritional values of these flavor boosters.

It's important to keep in mind that while these will add incredible flavor, it may not be the kind of flavor that you're used to. If your diet has been filled with processed meals, fast foods, or a lot of restaurant dishes, your palate has likely been programmed to think that only foods full of unhealthy amounts of fat, sugar, and salt are satisfying—but this couldn't be further from the truth. You can add savory, rich flavors to foods without relying heavily on this trio of additives. It might take a few days for your taste buds to wake up to the real flavor satisfaction found in natural herbs and spices and healthy fats, but once it does, you'll be in for an authentic palate-pleasing experience—one that doesn't harm your health or interfere with your weight loss goals.

Marinades and Poaching Broths

Many of the marinades in this section have suggested marinating times of four or more hours, but even just one hour of marinating time will add significant flavor.

Latin Marinade

Start to Finish: 10 minutes, plus 15 minutes to overnight for marinating
Make for: 1 pound pork loin or chicken
Yield: ⅓ cup

2 cloves garlic
1 tablespoon extra-virgin olive oil
1½ teaspoons chili powder
½ teaspoon ground cumin
1 teaspoon paprika
Pinch of ground cinnamon
1 teaspoon chopped oregano
1 teaspoon red wine vinegar
Salt and pepper to taste

1. In a bowl, mash garlic to a paste with a pinch of salt. Add remaining ingredients and stir to mix.
2. Place marinade in a leak-proof container or resealable bag. Add protein of your choice, pressing all the air out of the bag before you seal it so that the meat is in contact with the marinade. Chill in the refrigerator for 15 minutes to overnight.
3. Grill or sauté marinated meat.

Apple Cider Marinade

Start to Finish: 20 minutes, plus 15 minutes to overnight for marinating
Make for: 1 pound of pork loin or chicken
Yield: ½ cup

¼ cup apple cider
1 teaspoon cider vinegar
Pinch of ground cinnamon
½ tablespoon low-sodium soy sauce
1 teaspoon chopped sage
Salt and pepper to taste

1. Combine ingredients in a bowl; use a whisk to mix.
2. Place marinade in a leak-proof container or resealable bag. Add protein of your choice, pressing all the air out of the bag before you seal it so that the meat is in contact with the marinade. Chill in the refrigerator for 15 minutes to overnight.
3. Grill or sauté marinated meat.

Asian Herb Marinade

Start to Finish: 25 minutes, plus 4 to 24 hours for marinating
Make for: 2 pounds pork, chicken, or salmon
Yield: 1½ cups

¼ cup lightly packed fresh cilantro
⅓ cup minced fresh ginger
⅓ cup lightly packed fresh mint leaves
5 cloves garlic, halved
½ fresh serrano chili pepper, seeded and cut up*
½ tablespoon toasted sesame oil
1 tablespoon lime juice
½ teaspoon freshly ground black pepper
¼ teaspoon kosher salt

---

* Because hot chili peppers contain oils that can burn your skin and eyes, wear rubber or plastic gloves when working with them.

1. Combine all ingredients in a food processor. Cover and process to a thick paste, scraping down side of bowl as necessary.
2. To use as a marinade, spread over pork tenderloin, chicken breast halves, or salmon steaks. Cover and chill in the refrigerator for 4 to 24 hours.
3. Grill or roast pork; grill or broil chicken or salmon.

Cooking tip: You can place the marinade in a freezer container, seal, label, and freeze for up to three months. Thaw before using.

Chermoula Marinade

Start to Finish: 10 minutes, plus 8 to 24 hours for marinating
Make for: 3 to 4 pounds fish, poultry, beef, or pork
Yield: 1 cup

1½ tablespoons extra-virgin olive oil
⅓ cup lemon juice
⅓ cup chopped fresh flat-leaf parsley
⅓ cup chopped fresh cilantro
2 cloves garlic, minced
½ tablespoon paprika
⅓ teaspoon ground cumin
¼ teaspoon kosher salt
⅓ teaspoon cayenne pepper
¼ teaspoon freshly ground black pepper

1. In a medium bowl, whisk together all ingredients until combined.
2. To use as a marinade, place fish steaks, chicken breast halves, turkey breast tenderloins, beef steaks, or boneless pork chops in a resealable plastic bag; pour lemon juice mixture over. Seal bag and turn to coat fish, poultry, or meat. Chill in the refrigerator for 8 to 24 hours.
3. Grill or broil fish, poultry, or meat.

Chipotle Lime Marinade

Start to Finish: 15 minutes, plus 1 hour for marinating
Make for: 1 pound chicken, beef, or pork
Yield: ¾ cup

¼ cup lime juice
2 tablespoons chipotle peppers in adobo sauce (canned)
1 tablespoon ground coriander
Pinch of cumin seeds
4 teaspoons extra-virgin olive oil
⅛ teaspoon kosher salt

1. Combine all ingredients in a blender or food processor. Blend until smooth.
2. To use as a marinade, place chicken, beef, or pork in a resealable plastic bag; pour marinade mixture over. Seal bag and turn to coat. Chill in the refrigerator for up to 1 hour.
3. Grill or roast pork or beef; grill or broil chicken.

Cooking tip: If you want a spicier marinade, adjust the heat by using more of the chipotle peppers than the sauce.

Mediterranean Herb Marinade

Start to Finish: 20 minutes, plus 4 to 24 hours for marinating
Make for: 1 pound of pork, chicken, or salmon
Yield: ¾ cup

½ cup lightly packed fresh flat-leaf parsley
4 teaspoons extra-virgin olive oil
2 tablespoons fresh rosemary leaves
1 tablespoon fresh thyme leaves
1 tablespoon coarsely chopped fresh sage
1 tablespoon finely shredded lemon peel
5 cloves garlic, halved
½ teaspoon crushed red pepper
¼ teaspoon kosher salt
¼ teaspoon freshly ground black pepper

1. In a food processor, combine all ingredients. Cover and process to a thick paste, scraping down side of bowl as necessary.
2. To use as a marinade, spread over pork tenderloin, chicken breast halves, or salmon steaks. Cover and chill in the refrigerator for 4 to 24 hours.
3. Grill or roast pork; grill or broil chicken or salmon.

Cooking tip: You can place the marinade in a freezer container; seal, label, and freeze for up to 3 months. Thaw before using.

Spanish Marinade

Start to Finish: 10 minutes, plus 15 minutes to overnight for marinating
Make for: 1 pound of pork loin or chicken breasts
Yield: About ⅓ cup

1 clove garlic, mashed to a paste
1 tablespoon extra-virgin olive oil
½ teaspoon ground cumin, roasted
¼ teaspoon ground coriander, roasted
1 teaspoon Spanish paprika, smoked or plain
¼ teaspoon ground ginger
¼ teaspoon turmeric
¼ teaspoon ground black pepper
1 teaspoon lemon juice
Lemon zest

1. Mix ingredients together in a bowl.
2. To use as a marinade, place pork loin or chicken breasts in a resealable plastic bag; pour marinade mixture over. Seal bag and turn to coat pork or poultry. Chill in the refrigerator for 15 minutes to overnight.
3. Grill or sauté the meat.

Rubs for Meats, Poultry, and Fish

Coffee Rub

Start to Finish: 20 minutes, plus 30 minutes set time
Make for: 4 pounds of beef or pork
Yield: ½ cup

¼ cup chili powder
¼ cup coffee, finely ground
2 tablespoons Spanish paprika
2 tablespoons brown sugar
1 tablespoon ground coriander
½ teaspoon ground cinnamon
1 tablespoon kosher salt
1 tablespoon freshly ground black pepper
¼ teaspoon cayenne pepper

1. In a small bowl, stir together all ingredients.
2. Season meat with salt and pepper. Sprinkle evenly onto protein of your choice; rub in with your fingers. Let sit for 30 minutes prior to cooking.
3. Drizzle the meat with ½ to 1 tablespoon of oil.
4. Grill beef or pork.

Fresh Herb Rub

Start to Finish: 5 minutes
Make for: 2 pounds pork, poultry, or fish
Yield: ⅓ cup

1 tablespoon chopped fresh thyme, or ¾ teaspoon crushed dried thyme
1 tablespoon chopped fresh sage, or ¾ teaspoon crushed dried sage
1 tablespoon chopped fresh rosemary, or ¾ teaspoon crushed dried rosemary
2 cloves garlic, minced
1½ teaspoons coarsely ground black pepper

1 teaspoon kosher salt
½ teaspoon crushed red pepper

1. In a small bowl, stir together all ingredients.
2. Sprinkle evenly onto protein of your choice; rub in with your fingers.
3. Grill or broil pork, poultry, or fish.

Jamaican Jerk Rub

Start to Finish: 5 minutes, plus 30 minutes set time
Make for: 1 pound boneless pork chops, chicken breast halves, or turkey breast tenderloin
Yield: 1 cup

½ cup coarsely chopped onion
2 tablespoons lime juice
1 teaspoon crushed red pepper
½ teaspoon kosher salt
¼ teaspoon ground allspice
¼ teaspoon curry powder
¼ teaspoon freshly ground black pepper
⅛ teaspoon crushed dried thyme
⅛ teaspoon ground ginger
2 cloves garlic, quartered

1. Add all ingredients to blender. Cover and blend until smooth.
2. Sprinkle evenly onto protein of your choice; rub in with your fingers. Cover and chill in the refrigerator for 30 minutes.
3. Grill or broil pork or poultry.

Mustard-Peppercorn Rub

Start to Finish: 5 minutes, plus 15 minutes to 4 hours for refrigerating
Make for: 3 pounds boneless beef steaks, boneless pork chops, or boneless lamb chops
Yield: ⅓ cup

1 tablespoon prepared coarse-grain brown mustard
2 teaspoons extra-virgin olive oil

2 teaspoons cracked black peppercorns
2 teaspoons chopped fresh tarragon, or ½ teaspoon crushed dried tarragon
1 teaspoon kosher salt

1. In a small bowl, stir together all ingredients.
2. Sprinkle evenly onto protein of your choice; rub in with your fingers.
3. Cover and chill in the refrigerator for 15 minutes to 4 hours.
4. Grill or broil meat.

South American Spice Rub

Start to Finish: 5 minutes, plus 10 minutes set time
Make for: 1 pound lean protein of your choice (chicken, fish, beef, or pork)
Yield: ⅓ cup

1 tablespoon sweet paprika
1 tablespoon chili powder
1 teaspoon ground cumin
1 teaspoon oregano
1 teaspoon brown sugar
Pinch of cayenne pepper

1. Combine all ingredients together in a small bowl.
2. Season meat first with salt and pepper. Let sit for 10 minutes.
3. Sprinkle meat with spice mixture.
4. Grill or sauté.

Indian Spice Rub

Start to Finish: 5 minutes, plus 10 minutes set time
Make for: 1 pound lean protein of your choice (chicken, fish, beef, or pork)
Yield: ⅓ cup

1 tablespoon ground cumin
1 tablespoon curry powder
1 tablespoon chili powder

¼ tablespoon ground allspice
¼ tablespoon ground cinnamon
¼ teaspoon cayenne pepper
⅛ teaspoon salt
½ tablespoon ground black pepper

1. Combine all ingredients together in a small bowl.
2. Season meat first with salt and pepper. Let sit for 10 minutes.
3. Sprinkle meat with spice mixture.
4. Grill or sauté.

California Herb Rub

Start to Finish: 5 minutes, plus 10 minutes set time
Make for: 1 pound lean protein of your choice (chicken, fish, beef, or pork)
Yield: ⅓ cup

1 bay leaf
½ tablespoon summer savory
1 teaspoon dried basil
½ tablespoon dried thyme
½ tablespoon dried marjoram
½ tablespoon fennel seeds
½ teaspoon sage
½ teaspoon dried mint
½ teaspoon dried rosemary

1. Crumble and combine all the herbs together in a small bowl. Blend well.
2. Season meat first with salt and pepper. Let sit for 10 minutes.
3. Sprinkle meat with spice mixture.
4. Grill or sauté.

Spanish Rub

Start to Finish: 5 minutes, plus 10 minutes set time
Make for: 1 pound meat
Yield: ⅓ cup

½ tablespoon thyme
1 tablespoon ground cumin
1 tablespoon paprika
½ tablespoon red chili flakes
1 bay leaf
1 tablespoon parsley
½ teaspoon freshly ground black pepper

1. Crumble and combine all the herbs together in a small bowl. Blend well.
2. Season meat first with salt and pepper. Let sit for 10 minutes.
3. Sprinkle meat with spice mixture.
4. Grill or sauté.

Cooking Methods

The Love Diet recipes you'll find in the next chapter use several cooking methods with which you might be familiar, including grilling, baking, and roasting. Here, we provide a basic introduction to two flavor-boosting methods you may not use as often, poaching and steaming, which we encourage you to try during the Seven Stages. These methods are ideal if you're short on time—plus they're simple to use, even for a beginner cook.

Poaching

Poaching is a gentle cooking method that relies upon moist heat to cook foods. Foods are cooked in liquid that's been heated to a relatively low temperature, between 180°F and 185°F (because this is a gentle cooking method, you don't want the liquid to reach boiling temperatures). You've probably heard of or tried poached eggs, but you can poach everything from chicken and fish to fruits and vegetables. Let's take a look at how it's done.

We're going to focus on shallow poaching foods, which is the most common form of poaching and requires that you only partially submerge your ingredients in liquid. This method is ideal for smaller, individually portioned items such as chicken breasts, fish fillets, and beef tenderloins. You can use chicken or vegetable broths or vinegar as your poaching liquid, and then add herbs and spices to create a flavorful broth. A favorite poaching combination for seafood is fresh dill, basil, whole coriander seeds, and a squeeze of fresh lemon juice added to broth or water.

Since you want to use both steam and the liquid to cook your foods, the most important element with this method of cooking is that you use a lid to trap the steam and heat in the pan. Resist lifting the lid too soon—you'll release precious heat and get a warm steam bath to the face!

HOW TO SHALLOW POACH FOODS

1. Add herbs and spices or other flavoring ingredients to a wide shallow pan or frying pan with a tight-fitting lid.
2. Add your lean protein and the poaching liquid; fish, chicken, poultry, or beef should be placed in just enough liquid to come approximately halfway up the sides.
3. Bring the liquid to a simmer.
4. Cover your pan with the lid.
5. Simmer for approximately 20 minutes on low heat or until the lean protein is fully cooked and tender.
6. As the food is poaching, periodically skim the surface of the liquid as necessary (2 to 3 times total) to help the dish develop attractive colors and keep the broth from becoming too cloudy.
7. Remove your main ingredient and keep it warm.
8. Plate your food and serve with a drizzle of the poaching liquid.

BEST FOODS FOR POACHING

Shallow poaching is best suited for boneless, naturally tender meat, poultry, or fish that is single-serving size, sliced, or diced such as:

- Chicken
- Smaller and thinner cuts of beef and pork
- Fish and shellfish
- Fruits and vegetables
- Eggs

BEST COOKING LIQUIDS FOR POACHING

The cooking liquid will enhance your foods with flavor and serve as a delicious sauce (see the liquid used in the Fish Poached in the Spicy Chipotle Broth recipe as an example). Start with these liquids:

- Low-sodium broth
- Vinegar

BEST SPICES, HERBS, AND BROTH ADDITIONS

- Shallots
- Fennel
- Lemongrass
- Vegetables such as carrots, parsnips, or capers
- Herbs such as parsley, cilantro, rosemary, basil, tarragon, or a bay leaf
- Spices such as coriander, saffron, curry blends, or pepper
- Citrus zest

Steaming

Steaming cooks food by surrounding it with a vapor bath. Just like with poaching, you'll need to use a lid, but unlike with poaching, you will want to make sure to keep foods out of and above your cooking liquid instead of in it. This can be done simply by using a steamer basket, which you can find online or in any general cooking store.

HOW TO STEAM FOODS

1. Bring your herb-infused broth to a boil in a pot (the amount of liquid required depends on how long the food item will take to cook; the shorter the cooking time, the less liquid is needed).
2. Add the food item in a single layer to the steamer basket.
3. Cover the pot.
4. Steam the food to the correct doneness.
5. Serve the food immediately with the appropriate sauce and garnish.

BEST FOODS FOR STEAMING

- All vegetables
- Shellfish
- Meats, fish, and poultry

BEST COOKING LIQUIDS FOR STEAMING

- Water, especially if it has been infused with seasonings, herbs, or spices
- Broth

BEST SPICES TO ADD TO STEAMING LIQUID

- Herbs such as parsley, cilantro, rosemary, basil, tarragon, or a bay leaf
- Spices such as coriander, saffron, curry blends, or pepper
- Garlic
- Citrus rinds

CHAPTER 15

The Love Diet Recipes

Welcome to the Love Diet recipes. We hope you'll turn to this section often throughout the program and that it will help you discover how incredible healthful foods can taste—and how easily they can be prepared! Whether you're a beginning or experienced cook, it's important to consider the gift you're giving yourself when you make your own meals—there's a reason you hear home cooks use the phrase "made with love."

All of the recipes included here have been organized into specific categories and noted with information indicating in which stages you can enjoy them. You'll find recipes for Vinaigrettes, Salads and Chilies, Beef, Poultry, and Pork Dishes, Breakfast Dishes, and Side Dishes, Dips, and Sauces. With the exception of the vinaigrettes, which you can have during the entire Seven Stages, each category's recipes are featured in the order in which you'll be able to include them in your diet—meaning recipes for the earlier stages will appear first and those for the later stages will appear last. This will make it easy for you to start from the front and work your way back as you progress through the program.

Have fun discovering new recipes and foods, and don't be afraid to make modifications if you'd like—just be sure to refer to your nutrition guidelines for each stage that you are currently in.

Vinaigrettes

Greek Vinaigrette

Start to Finish: 15 minutes
Stages: 1–7
Yield: About ⅓ cup

1 tablespoon red wine vinegar
1 tablespoon lemon juice
3 tablespoons extra-virgin olive oil
1 tablespoon chopped fresh oregano, or ½ tablespoon dry oregano
Dash of kosher salt
Dash of freshly ground black pepper

1. In a small bowl, combine vinegar and lemon juice.
2. Add oil in a thin, steady stream, whisking constantly until combined. Stir in oregano, kosher salt, and pepper.
3. Use immediately or cover and chill for up to 3 days before using. If chilled, let stand at room temperature for 30 minutes; whisk before using.

Nutrition Facts per Serving: calories 73, fat 8 g, carbohydrate 0 g, protein 0 g, sodium 24 mg.

Pesto Vinaigrette

Start to Finish: 10 minutes
Stages: 1–7
Yield: ¾ cup

1 cup packed fresh basil leaves
⅓ cup extra-virgin olive oil
1 tablespoon pine nuts, toasted
¼ cup white wine vinegar
½ teaspoon kosher salt
¼ teaspoon freshly ground black pepper

1. In a food processor, combine basil leaves, oil, and nuts. Cover and pulse to a coarse puree.
2. Transfer mixture to a small bowl. Whisk in vinegar, kosher salt, and pepper.

Nutrition Facts per Serving: calories 80, fat 8 g, carbohydrate 1 g, protein 1 g, sodium 81 mg.

Red Wine Vinaigrette

Start to Finish: 10 minutes
Stages: 1–7
Yield: About ⅓ cup

2 tablespoons red wine vinegar
1½ teaspoons Dijon mustard
2 tablespoons extra-virgin olive oil
⅛ teaspoon kosher salt
⅛ teaspoon freshly ground black pepper

1. Pour vinegar into a small bowl.
2. Whisk in mustard. Add oil in a thin, steady stream, whisking constantly until combined. Stir in kosher salt and pepper.
3. Use immediately or cover and chill for up to 3 days before using. If chilled, let stand at room temperature about 30 minutes; whisk before using.

Nutrition Facts per Serving: calories 51, fat 5 g, carbohydrate 1 g, protein 0 g, sodium 85 mg.

Simple Lemon Vinaigrette

Start to Finish: 10 minutes
Stages: 1–7
Yield: ½ cup

¼ cup lemon juice
¼ cup extra-virgin olive oil
Salt and pepper to taste

Combine all ingredients. Whisk well.

Variation: Replace lemon juice with lime juice.

Nutrition Facts per Serving: calories 30, fat 3 g, carbohydrate 0 g, protein 0 g, sodium 32 mg.

Soy Sesame Vinaigrette

Start to Finish: 10 minutes
Stages: 1–7
Yield: ½ cup

4 tablespoons low-sodium soy sauce
1 tablespoon rice vinegar
½ tablespoon lemon juice
1 tablespoon minced or grated ginger
1 clove garlic, chopped
2 teaspoons sesame oil
Salt and pepper to taste

Combine all ingredients. Whisk well.

Cooking tip: Use a microplane to grate the ginger; it allows you to grate the pulp from the ginger root and leave the stringy, fibrous core behind.

Nutrition Facts per Serving: calories 22, fat 1 g, carbohydrate 1 g, protein 1.5 g, sodium 300 mg.

Balsamic Vinaigrette

Start to Finish: 10 minutes
Stages: 1–7
Yield: 1 cup

½ cup low-sodium chicken broth
¼ cup balsamic vinegar
1 tablespoon chopped fresh basil, or 1 teaspoon crushed dried basil
Dash of kosher salt
⅓ cup extra-virgin olive oil
Kosher salt (optional)

ARE YOU PEELING AND SELECTING AVOCADOS THE RIGHT WAY?*

Avocados contribute carotenoids, naturally occurring pigments with antioxidant properties found in fruits and vegetables. In California Avocados, the greatest concentration of beneficial carotenoids is in the dark green fruit of the avocado closest to the peel. The best way to get to this nutrient-rich fruit directly under the peel is to cut the avocado in half lengthwise around the seed, then turn it a quarter and cut in half lengthwise again (giving you four quarters). Remove the seed gently with your fingertips and then—this is the key part—peel the skin away from the avocado to help ensure you get the most of the nutritious outer layer. A video of this technique can be seen at: CaliforniaAvocado.com/how-tos/how-to-choose-and-use-an-avocado#cut-cac. To select an avocado, look for large (about 8 ounces), ripe fruit. An avocado that yields to gentle pressure is ideal and should be eaten within two to three days. Once cut, sprinkle with lemon or lime juice and cover in plastic wrap, pressing the plastic wrap tightly around the avocado.

*Source: California Avocado Commission (CaliforniaAvocado.com)

1. In a small bowl, combine chicken broth, vinegar, basil, and a dash of kosher salt.
2. Add oil in a thin, steady stream, whisking constantly until combined.
3. If desired, season to taste with additional kosher salt.
4. Use immediately or cover and chill for up to 1 week before using. If chilled, let stand at room temperature for 30 minutes; whisk before serving.

Nutrition Facts per Serving: calories 33, fat 3 g, carbohydrate 1 g, protein 0 g, sodium 38 mg.

Salads and Chilies

Avocado Tuna Salad

Start to Finish: 15 minutes
Stages: 1–7
Yield: 3 servings

1 12-ounce can chunk light tuna in water, drained and flaked
⅛ large, ripe Fresh California Avocado, peeled, seeded and cut into chunks

¼ cup reduced-fat mayonnaise
3 teaspoons lemon juice
1½ teaspoons chopped fresh oregano, or ¼ teaspoon dry oregano

Combine all ingredients in a medium bowl and mix until blended well.

Nutrition Facts per Serving: calories 173, fat 6.5 g, carbohydrate 5 g, protein 26.5 g, sodium 600 mg.

Asian Chopped Chicken Salad

Start to Finish: 35 minutes
Stages: 2–7
Yield: 4 servings

Nonstick olive oil cooking spray
16 ounces cooked lean chicken, shredded or sliced very thin
¼ cup snow peas, blanched and chopped
¼ cup chopped red and yellow peppers
1 cup chopped red leaf lettuce
¼ cup sliced cucumber—peeled, cut in half lengthwise, seeded, and sliced thin
1 tablespoon chopped toasted almonds
2 tablespoons Soy Sesame Vinaigrette (page 210)

1. Coat 4 6-ounce coffee cups with nonstick cooking spray.
2. Equally divide and layer ingredients in each cup in the following order: chicken, snow peas, bell pepper, lettuce, and cucumber.
3. Cover tops with plastic wrap and firmly press mixture into cups with a soup can or similar object slightly smaller than diameter of cup.
4. To serve, invert salads onto 4 salad plates; carefully lift off cups. Sprinkle salads with almonds; drizzle with vinaigrette.

Cooking tip: For ease of preparation, pour a quarter of the vinaigrette in the bottom of each cup; then start layering ingredients on top, pressing down slightly to compress so the salad holds together. Cover and refrigerate overnight if desired. When you invert the cups, the vinaigrette will drizzle down onto the rest of the ingredients.

Nutrition Facts per Serving: calories 320, fat 12 g, carbohydrate 9 g, protein 43 g, sodium 430 mg.

Broccoli Salad with Sun-Dried Tomatoes

Start to Finish: 20 minutes
Stages: 2–7
Yield: 4 servings

1 pound broccoli florets and stems
1 ounce sun-dried tomatoes (soft, julienned, not packed in oil)
1 ounce sliced almonds, toasted
2 scallions, sliced thin on a bias
1 tablespoon basil, julienned
5 tablespoons Red Wine Vinaigrette (page 209)
Salt and pepper to taste

1. Fill a 2-quart pot with water. Bring to a boil. Add 1 tablespoon salt and bring back to a boil.
2. Add the broccoli florets and cook until crisp-tender, about 2 minutes. Place in ice water to shock. Let cool 3 to 5 minutes; drain well.
3. Peel and trim the broccoli stems. Cut stems in half lengthwise; then slice ⅛ inch thin on a bias.
4. In a bowl, combine the broccoli florets and stems with the remaining ingredients. Toss well.

Cooking tip: To keep the salad from discoloring, add the vinaigrette just before serving.

Variation: Replace broccoli with cauliflower.

Nutrition Facts per Serving: calories 150, fat 8 g, carbohydrate 15 g, protein 5 g, sodium 550 mg.

Super-Quick Dinner Salad

Start to Finish: 15 minutes
Stages: 2–7
Yield: 4 servings

1 bag prewashed mixed salad greens or baby spinach
2 tablespoons chopped green onions or red onions
½ cup chopped Roma, cherry, or other in-season tomato
¼ cup Newman's Own Light Balsamic vinaigrette dressing
Freshly ground black pepper

1. Place the salad greens, chopped onion, and tomatoes in a large salad bowl.
2. Drizzle vinaigrette dressing on top and toss lightly.
3. Top it off with freshly ground black pepper, if desired.

Other ingredient ideas: 1 16-ounce can artichoke hearts in water, drained and cut into quarters; red bell pepper, cut into strips; grated carrot or red cabbage; sliced radishes; cucumber, peeled, seeded, and sliced; 2 tablespoons grated Parmesan cheese; 5–6 ounces leftover cooked salmon, chicken, or shrimp.

Nutrition Facts per Serving*: calories 60, fat 1 g, carbohydrate 11 g, protein 2 g, sodium 145 mg.

Grilled Asparagus Salad

Start to Finish: 20 minutes
Stages: 3–7
Yield: 2 servings

12 ounces fresh asparagus (thick spears), trimmed
2 tablespoons extra-virgin olive oil
¼ teaspoon kosher salt
⅛ teaspoon freshly ground black pepper
3 tablespoons lemon juice
2 hard-boiled eggs, peeled and chopped
1 tablespoon grated Parmesan cheese

* Nutritional analysis does not include additional ingredient ideas.

1. In a large bowl, toss asparagus spears with 1 tablespoon olive oil. Sprinkle with kosher salt and pepper.
2. For a charcoal grill, place asparagus spears crosswise on the rack of an uncovered grill directly over medium coals. Grill for 5 to 7 minutes, or until asparagus is crisp-tender and slightly charred all over, turning occasionally. For a gas grill, preheat grill. Reduce heat to medium. Place asparagus spears crosswise on grill rack over heat. Cover and grill as above.
3. To serve, transfer grilled asparagus to serving platter. Drizzle with lemon juice and remaining 1 tablespoon olive oil. Sprinkle with chopped eggs and Parmesan cheese. Serve immediately or cover and chill for up to 24 hours.

Broiler method: Place asparagus on the unheated rack of a broiler pan. Broil 4 to 5 inches from the heat for 5 to 7 minutes, or until asparagus is crisp-tender, turning once halfway through broiling.

Variation: Asparagus with Pesto Vinaigrette: Stir in 1 tablespoon pesto with the lemon juice and olive oil.

Nutrition Facts per Serving: 150 calories, protein 5 g, fat 8 g, carbohydrate 15 g, sodium 550 mg.

California Chicken Salad in Lettuce Cups

Start to Finish: 30 minutes, plus 1 to 24 hours for marinating
Stages: 3–7
Yield: 4 servings

4 cups coarsely shredded cooked chicken breast (about 1¼ pounds)
1 15-ounce jar roasted red and yellow bell peppers, drained and cut into strips
1 6-ounce jar marinated artichoke hearts, drained and coarsely chopped
¼ cup thinly sliced red onion
2 tablespoons chopped fresh flat-leaf parsley
2 tablespoons capers, rinsed and drained
Simple Lemon Vinaigrette (page 209)

4 large butterhead (Bibb or Boston) lettuce leaves
¾ cup (2 ounces) shaved Parmesan cheese

1. In a large bowl, combine chicken, roasted bell peppers, artichoke hearts, red onion, parsley, and capers.
2. Drizzle with lemon vinaigrette; toss gently to coat. Cover and chill for 1 to 24 hours.
3. To serve, place a lettuce leaf on each of 4 dinner plates. Spoon chicken salad onto lettuce leaves. Sprinkle with Parmesan cheese.

Nutrition Facts per Serving: calories 303, fat 15 g, carbohydrate 8 g, protein 35 g, sodium 466 mg.

Chopped Salad with Blue Cheese Dressing*

Start to Finish: 30 minutes
Stages: 3–7
Yield: 4 servings

6 cups chopped Romaine lettuce
2 cups sliced cucumber
1 cup diced plum tomato
1 cup sliced celery
1 cup sliced radishes
1 cup diced red bell pepper
½ cup diced carrot
½ cup thinly sliced green onions
¼ cup chopped fresh Italian flat-leaf parsley
3 tablespoons capers, drained
1 teaspoon dried oregano

FOR DRESSING:

⅓ cup low-fat buttermilk
¼ cup (1 ounce) crumbled blue cheese
1 tablespoon light mayonnaise
1 tablespoon red wine vinegar

* To make this dish a complete meal, add 4 to 6 ounces lean protein per serving. Specific serving size will depend upon the stage you are in and whether you are male or female.

1 teaspoon Worcestershire sauce
¼ teaspoon freshly ground black pepper
Pinch of kosher salt

1. To prepare salad, combine first 11 ingredients in a large bowl.
2. To prepare dressing, combine buttermilk and remaining ingredients in a small bowl, stirring with a whisk.
3. Just before serving, drizzle salad with dressing and toss gently to coat.

Nutrition Facts per Serving: calories 110, fat 4.5 g, carbohydrate 16 g, protein 6 g, sodium 150 mg.

Old-Fashioned Chicken Salad

Start to Finish: 35 minutes
Stages: 4–7
Yield: 6 servings

1 pound cooked chicken breast, cubed
2 Granny Smith apples, cored and chopped
1 cup peeled and chopped celery
½ cup chopped scallions
2 tablespoons chopped fresh flat-leaf parsley
¼ cup nonfat plain yogurt
¼ cup white wine vinegar
3 tablespoons low-fat or fat-free mayonnaise
Pinch of kosher salt
¼ teaspoon freshly ground black pepper
¼ cup sliced almonds, toasted
6 cups torn mixed salad greens

1. In a large bowl combine chicken, apples, celery, scallions, and parsley.
2. In a small bowl, combine yogurt, white wine vinegar, mayonnaise, kosher salt, and pepper.
3. Add to chicken mixture. Stir in sliced almonds.
4. Divide greens among 6 serving plates; top with chicken mixture.

Nutrition Facts per Serving: calories 200, fat 10 g, carbohydrate 11 g, protein 26 g, sodium 288 mg.

Mixed Greens, Pear, and Low-Fat Blue Cheese Salad*

Start to Finish: 15 minutes
Stages: 4–7
Yield: 4 servings

2 lemon wedges
1 pear, sliced into wedges
2½ cups mixed baby greens
¼ cup chopped pecans, toasted
½ cup (2 ounces) crumbled reduced-fat blue cheese
4 tablespoons Trader Joe's Cranberry, Walnut & Gorgonzola Dressing

1. Squeeze lemon wedges over pear wedges; set aside.
2. In a large bowl, toss the salad greens, pecans, blue cheese, and pear slices.
3. Serve with a side of 1 tablespoon of dressing each.

Nutrition Facts per Serving: calories 184, fat 12 g, carbohydrate 11 g, protein 9 g, sodium 175 mg.

Asian Asparagus-and-Orange Salad

Start to Finish: 20 minutes
Stages: 4–7
Yield: 5 servings

1 medium orange, tennis ball size
½ tablespoon extra-virgin olive oil
3 cups diagonally sliced asparagus (about 1 pound)
1 small garlic clove, thinly sliced
1 teaspoon low-sodium soy sauce
⅛ teaspoon dark sesame oil
½ tablespoon sesame seeds, toasted
Napa (Chinese) cabbage leaves (optional)

1. Peel and section oranges over a bowl. Juice one section of orange, or enough to give you 1 teaspoon of juice; reserve juice. Set remaining sections aside, discarding membranes.

* To make this dish a complete meal, add 3 to 6 ounces of lean protein and ½ cup berries per serving. Specific protein serving size will depend upon the stage you are in and whether you are male or female.

2. Heat olive oil in a large skillet over medium-high heat. Add asparagus and garlic; sauté 5 minutes and remove from pan.
3. In a small bowl, combine soy sauce and sesame oil; pour over asparagus mixture, tossing well. Cool to room temp.
4. Stir in sesame seeds, orange sections, and 1 teaspoon orange juice.
5. Serve on cabbage leaves, if desired.

Nutrition Facts per Serving: calories 60, fat 2 g, carbohydrate 8 g, protein 3 g, sodium 175 mg.

Onion, Orange, and Olive Salad with Tuna*

Start to Finish: 30 minutes
Stages: 4–7
Yield: 6 servings

4 navel oranges, peeled and cut crosswise into thin slices
½ cup thinly sliced onion
1 6-ounce can albacore tuna in water, drained
¼ cup sliced ripe olives
2 tablespoons white wine vinegar
2 tablespoons orange juice
1 tablespoon extra-virgin olive oil
¼ teaspoon cumin seeds
⅛ teaspoon crushed red pepper
1 garlic clove, crushed

1. Arrange orange slices and onion slices on a serving platter and top with tuna and olive slices.
2. Combine the vinegar and remaining ingredients in a small bowl and stir with a whisk until well blended.
3. Drizzle vinegar mixture over salad.

Nutrition Facts per Serving: calories 120, fat 3 g, carbohydrate 14 g, protein 9 g, sodium 145 mg.

* To make this dish a complete meal, increase protein to 4 to 6 ounces lean protein per serving. Specific serving size will depend upon the stage you are in and whether you are male or female.

Roasted Pepper and Chickpea Salad

Start to Finish: 15 minutes
Stages: 6–7
Yield: 4 servings

½ cup vertically sliced red onion
⅓ cup minced fresh cilantro
2 tablespoons fresh lemon juice
1 tablespoon extra-virgin olive oil
½ teaspoon Hungarian sweet paprika
¼ teaspoon kosher salt
¼ teaspoon freshly ground black pepper
3 jarred roasted red bell peppers, peeled and cut into thin strips
1 garlic clove, crushed
1 15-ounce can chickpeas (garbanzo beans), drained

Combine all ingredients in medium bowl and toss salad well.

Nutrition Facts per Serving: calories 160, fat 5 g, carbohydrate 23 g, protein 6 g, sodium 165 mg.

Balsamic Bean Salad

Start to Finish: 15 minutes, plus up to 4 hours for marinating
Stages: 6–7
Yield: 7 servings

1 cup frozen cut green beans
1 16-ounce can kidney beans
1 15-ounce can garbanzo beans
1 cup diced red onion
½ cup balsamic vinegar
¼ cup water
2 tablespoons Dijon mustard
1 tablespoon extra-virgin olive oil
1 teaspoon dried thyme
¼ teaspoon kosher salt
¼ teaspoon ground white pepper
2 cloves garlic, minced

1. Combine first 3 ingredients in a colander; rinse and drain.
2. Combine onion and remaining ingredients in a bowl. Add bean mixture, tossing gently to coat.
3. Cover and marinate in refrigerator up to 4 hours (optional), stirring occasionally.
4. Serve with a slotted spoon.

Nutrition Facts per Serving: calories 150, fat 4 g, carbohydrate 28 g, protein 8 g, sodium 50 mg.

Crab Salad with White Beans and Gourmet Greens

Start to Finish: 30 minutes
Stages: 6–7
Yield: 6 servings

⅓ cup chopped yellow bell pepper
⅓ cup chopped red onion
¼ cup chopped celery
2 tablespoons white wine vinegar
1 tablespoon fresh lemon juice
1 tablespoon extra-virgin olive oil
¼ teaspoon kosher salt
⅛ teaspoon Tabasco hot sauce
2 6-ounce cans lump crabmeat, drained, or 12 ounces fresh cooked crabmeat
1 16-ounce can cannellini beans or other white beans, rinsed and drained
6 cups torn gourmet salad greens

1. Combine first 10 ingredients; toss gently.
2. Cover and chill 20 minutes. Serve over greens.

Nutrition Facts per Serving: calories 150, fat 4 g, carbohydrate 13 g, protein 17 g, sodium 375 mg.

Toasted Quinoa Pilaf

Start to Finish: 30 minutes
Stage: 7
Yield: 8 servings

GLUTEN-FREE

2 tablespoons extra-virgin olive oil
2 cups quinoa, rinsed, drained well
1 cup diced onion
1 tablespoon chopped garlic
2 teaspoons chopped thyme
2½ cups water or broth
Salt and pepper to taste

1. Heat a small saucepan over medium heat. Add olive oil and quinoa. Toast the quinoa, stirring occasionally. It will start to pop like popcorn and have a slightly nutty aroma.
2. Add onion, garlic, and thyme; stir until aromatic.
3. Add water; bring to a simmer.
4. Season with salt and pepper. Reduce heat to low, cover tightly, and cook for 15 minutes.
5. Remove from heat, let sit for 4 minutes, and fluff with a fork.

Cooking tips: Quinoa has a natural coating on the outside called saposin, which can have a bitter taste. To reduce some of the bitterness, rinse quinoa in water first. Let it drain and dry for at least a few minutes before toasting; if the grain is wet, will be more difficult to toast.

Quinoa can also be toasted by spreading it on a sheet pan and placing in a 350°F oven for 5 to 10 minutes, stirring periodically.

It is important to let the grain sit for a few minutes once it is removed from the heat. This allows the grain to settle and slightly firm up. If you stir it immediately after it has finished cooking, it will mush up and become gummy.

Variations: Add 2 cups mushrooms sautéed with garlic. Or try adding ¼ cup chopped sun-dried tomatoes along with the garlic, onion, and thyme, and then 1 tablespoon basil, added to the quinoa once it is removed from heat.

Nutrition Facts per Serving: calories 100, fat 3 g, carbohydrate 16 g, protein 4 g, sodium 10 mg.

Chicken, Tomato, Basil, and Pasta Salad

Start to Finish: 20 minutes
Stage: 7
Yield: 4 servings

1 tablespoon extra-virgin olive oil
1 clove garlic, sliced
2 cups whole wheat penne pasta or Barilla Plus pasta, cooked
3 tablespoons red wine vinegar
2 cups seeded and diced tomatoes
1 pound chicken, cooked, shredded
1½ cups baby spinach, cut into 1-inch pieces
3 tablespoons capers, rinsed, roughly chopped
1 tablespoon chopped basil
2 scallions, chopped
Salt and pepper to taste

1. Place olive oil and garlic in a small pan. Cook over low heat until garlic is tender, about 5 minutes.
2. Place cooked penne in a bowl. Toss with 1 tablespoon of the vinegar. Add cooked garlic and oil.
3. Add tomatoes, chicken, spinach, capers, basil, and scallions. Add the remaining vinegar and toss well. Adjust seasoning with salt and pepper.

Nutrition Facts per Serving: calories 285, fat 10 g, carbohydrate 7 g, protein 45 g, sodium 310 mg.

Toasted Quinoa, Chicken, and Avocado Salad*

Start to Finish: 25 minutes
Stage: 7
Yield: 4 servings

GLUTEN-FREE

1 cup peeled, seeded, and diced cucumbers
2 cups quinoa, cooked
1 cup cooked and shredded chicken
1 cup seeded and diced red pepper
2 scallions, chopped
2 tablespoons chopped cilantro
4 tablespoons Simple Lemon Vinaigrette (page 209)
½ large, ripe Fresh California Avocado, peeled, seeded, and diced
Salt and pepper to taste

1. Place cucumbers in a bowl. Lightly season with salt and pepper. Let sit for 5 minutes. Drain.
2. Add quinoa, chicken, red pepper, scallions, and cilantro. Gently mix.
3. Add vinaigrette and adjust seasoning with salt and pepper. Fold in avocado.

Cooking tip: To avoid mushing the avocado, it should be the last thing added to the salad. Do not mix after it is added.

Nutrition Facts per Serving: calories 250, fat 13 g, carbohydrate 30 g, protein 14 g, sodium 89 mg.

Greek Salad with Grilled Shrimp

Start to Finish: 1 hour
Stage: 7
Yield: 4 servings

1 pound fresh or frozen large shrimp in shells, heads removed
2 cloves garlic, minced

* To make this dish a complete meal, increase protein to 4 to 6 ounces of lean protein per serving. Specific serving size will depend upon the stage you are in and whether you are male or female.

½ teaspoon finely shredded lemon peel
3 cups whole fresh baby spinach leaves
3 cups torn romaine
2 medium tomatoes, cut into thin wedges
⅓ cup red onion, thinly sliced
1 medium cucumber, quartered lengthwise and sliced ¼ inch thick
⅓ cup pitted kalamata olives
¼ cup radishes, thinly sliced
¼ cup (1 ounce) crumbled feta cheese
⅓ cup Greek Vinaigrette (page 208)
2 whole wheat pita bread rounds, halved crosswise

1. Thaw shrimp, if frozen. Peel and devein, leaving tails intact if desired. Rinse shrimp; pat dry with paper towels. In a small bowl, toss shrimp with garlic and lemon peel. Cover and chill for 30 minutes.
2. Meanwhile, in a large bowl combine spinach, romaine, tomatoes, cucumber, olives, red onion, and radishes; toss to combine. Set aside.
3. Thread shrimp onto 4 8-inch skewers, leaving ¼-inch space between pieces.
4. For a charcoal grill, place skewers on the greased rack of an uncovered grill directly over medium coals. Grill for 6 to 8 minutes or until shrimp are opaque, turning once halfway through grilling. For a gas grill, preheat grill. Reduce heat to medium. Place skewers on greased grill rack over heat. Cover and grill as above.
5. To serve, divide greens among four dinner plates. Sprinkle with feta cheese. Top with grilled shrimp. Drizzle with Greek Vinaigrette. Serve with pita bread.

Broiler method: Place skewers on the unheated rack of a broiler pan. Broil 4 inches from heat for 2 to 4 minutes or until shrimp are opaque, turning once halfway through broiling.

Cooking tip: If using wooden skewers, soak in enough water to cover for at least 1 hour before grilling.

Variation: Replace shrimp with ½-inch by 3-inch strips of boneless skinless chicken breasts.

Nutrition Facts per Serving: calories 369, fat 16 g, carbohydrate 29 g, protein 30 g, sodium 571 mg.

Slow Cooker White Bean Chicken Chili

Start to Finish: 5 to 10 hours, depending on slow cooker setting
Stages: 6–7
Yield: 6 servings

2 15-ounce cans Great Northern beans, drained and rinsed
20 ounces cooked chicken breasts, shredded
1 cup chopped onion
1½ cups chopped yellow, red, or green bell pepper
2 cloves garlic, minced
2 teaspoons cumin
½ teaspoon kosher salt
½ teaspoon dried oregano
3½ cups nonfat, low-sodium chicken broth (2 14-ounce cans)
Cayenne pepper to taste
4 tablespoons low-fat sour cream
1 cup (4 ounces) grated reduced-fat mozzarella cheese

1. In a slow cooker, combine all ingredients except cayenne pepper, sour cream, and cheese and cover. Cook on low for 8 to 10 hours, or on high for 4 to 5 hours.
2. Add cayenne pepper and stir. Ladle into bowls and top individual servings with ¼ cup shredded mozzarella and 1 tablespoon low-fat sour cream per serving, as garnish.

Nutrition Facts per Serving: calories 280, fat 4.5 g, carbohydrate 25 g, protein 39 g, sodium 500 mg.

Lentil Turkey Chili

Start to Finish: 1 hour, 15 minutes
Stages: 6–7
Yield: 6 servings

2 pounds ground lean turkey breast
1 pound lentils (about 2½ cups)
5 cups water
1 teaspoon kosher salt
1 16-ounce can tomatoes or tomato sauce
1 medium onion, chopped
1½ tablespoons chili powder
⅛ teaspoon garlic powder, or 1 clove garlic, minced

1. Brown the ground turkey meat over medium heat for approximately 8 minutes in same pot that will be used to make the chili.
2. Wash and drain lentils.
3. Add lentils, water, and salt to pot; bring to a boil. Reduce heat, cover, and boil gently for 30 minutes.
4. Add tomatoes or tomato sauce, onion, chili powder, and garlic or garlic powder; stir. Cover and boil gently for 30 more minutes.

Nutrition Facts per Serving: calories 510, fat 15 g, carbohydrate 53 g, protein 47 g, sodium 650 mg.

Beef, Poultry, and Pork Dishes

Grilled Chimichurri Flank Steak

Start to Finish: 1 hour, plus 1 to 24 hours for marinating
Stages: 1–7
Yield: 6 servings

1 pound flat iron or flank steak, thinly sliced
¼ cup red wine vinegar
2 tablespoons extra-virgin olive oil
¾ cup beef broth or water
½ cup chopped Italian parsley

2–3 cloves garlic, minced
3 tablespoons minced shallots
2 tablespoons chopped oregano
¾ teaspoon red chili flakes
1 teaspoon lemon juice
Salt to taste

1. Trim fat from meat. Score both sides of steak in a diamond pattern by making shallow cuts at 1-inch intervals. Place steak in a shallow dish; set aside.
2. In a small bowl, stir together remaining ingredients, using only up to 1 teaspoon salt, depending on the saltiness of the beef broth.
3. Spoon mixture evenly over both sides of steak; rub in with your fingers. Cover and marinate in the refrigerator for 1 to 24 hours.
4. Remove refrigerated meat at least 15 minutes prior to grilling to allow meat to reach room temperature.
5. For a charcoal grill, place meat on the rack of an uncovered grill directly over medium coals. Grill for 17 to 21 minutes or until medium doneness (160°F), turning once halfway through grilling. For a gas grill, preheat grill. Reduce heat to medium and place meat on grill rack over heat. Cover and grill as above.
6. Transfer grilled meat to a cutting board. Cover and let stand for 10 minutes.
7. To serve, slice very thinly across the grain.

Nutrition Facts per Serving: calories 233, fat 6 g, carbohydrate 12 g, protein 29 g, sodium 377 mg.

Herb-Marinated Flank Steak

Start to Finish: 1 hour, plus 1 to 24 hours for marinating
Stages: 1–7
Yield: 6 servings

1 1½- to 2-pound beef flank steak
¼ cup chopped fresh rosemary, or 1 tablespoon crushed dried rosemary

1 tablespoon chopped fresh oregano, or 1 teaspoon crushed dried oregano
3 cloves garlic, minced
1½ teaspoons paprika
1 teaspoon kosher salt
1 teaspoon crushed red pepper
1 teaspoon freshly ground black pepper
3 tablespoons extra-virgin olive oil

1. Trim fat from meat. Score both sides of steak in a diamond pattern by making shallow cuts at 1-inch intervals. Place steak in a shallow dish; set aside.
2. In a small bowl, stir together rosemary, oregano, garlic, paprika, kosher salt, crushed red pepper, and black pepper. Stir in the oil until combined.
3. Spoon herb mixture evenly over both sides of steak; rub in with your fingers. Cover and marinate in the refrigerator for 1 to 24 hours.
4. Remove refrigerated meat at least 15 minutes prior to grilling to allow meat to reach room temperature.
5. For a charcoal grill, place meat on the rack of an uncovered grill directly over medium coals. Grill for 17 to 21 minutes or until medium doneness (160°F), turning once halfway through grilling. For a gas grill, preheat grill. Reduce heat to medium. Place meat on grill rack over heat. Cover and grill as above.
6. Transfer grilled meat to a cutting board. Cover and let stand for 10 minutes.
7. To serve, slice very thinly across the grain.

Nutrition Facts per Serving: calories 183, fat 11 g, carbohydrate 1 g, protein 19 g, sodium 287 mg.

Cal-Asian Lettuce Wrap Burger*

Start to Finish: 15 minutes
Stages: 2-7
Yield: 4 servings

1 pound (90/10 lean to fat ratio) ground beef
2 cloves garlic, minced
1 teaspoon grated fresh ginger
1 tablespoon hoisin sauce
1 teaspoon low-sodium soy sauce
8 ounces shiitake mushrooms, stems removed, caps sliced ¼-inch thick
½ teaspoon toasted sesame oil
2 tablespoons extra-virgin olive oil, divided
1 large, ripe Fresh California Avocado, seeded, peeled, and sliced
½ cup finely julienned or shredded carrots
2 green onions, white and light green part only, thinly sliced
4 large butter lettuce leaves
Sriracha for serving (optional)

1. Combine the beef, garlic, ginger, hoisin sauce, and soy sauce in a bowl and mix well. Form into burger patties about ½-inch thick. Set aside.
2. Heat half of the olive oil in a large non-stick skillet over medium high heat. Add mushroom slices and sauté until golden, about 4–5 minutes. Remove from heat and transfer to a small bowl. Toss with the toasted sesame oil.
3. Heat the remaining olive oil in the pan over medium high heat. Add the burger patties and cook for 3 minutes, then flip and cook for an additional 3–4 minutes for medium-rare. Remove the patties from the pan.
4. Place each burger patty on a lettuce leaf. Top each with the mushrooms, avocado slices, carrots, green onions, and bean sprouts. Serve with Sriracha (optional).

---

* Recipe provided by California Avocado Commission. Copyright © 2015

Cooking tip: Large avocados are recommended for this recipe. A large avocado averages about 8 ounces. If using smaller or larger size avocados adjust the quantity accordingly. As with all fruits and vegetables, wash avocados before cutting.

Nutrition Information Per Serving: calories 380, fat 25 g, carbohydrate 16 g; protein 25 g; sodium 210 mg.

Roast Chicken

Start to Finish: 1½ hours
Stages: 1–7
Yield: 6 servings

2 tablespoons white wine
2 tablespoons extra-virgin olive oil
1 tablespoon Dijon mustard
2 tablespoons chopped rosemary
2–3 cloves garlic, chopped
Pepper to taste
1 whole chicken, giblets and excess fat removed

1. Place a shallow roasting pan with a rack in the oven. Preheat oven to 375°F.
2. In a small bowl, combine olive oil, wine, mustard, rosemary, and garlic. Season with pepper.
3. Gently loosen the skin from the breast and legs of the chicken, being careful not to tear the skin. Rub ¾ of the rosemary mixture underneath the skin of the chicken. Rub the remaining ¼ all over the skin.
4. Place the chicken on the rack in the roasting pan in the oven. Roast 50 to 60 minutes until the juice runs clear, or until the chicken is 165°F at the thigh or approximately 160°F at the breast.
5. Let rest in a warm place for 15 minutes prior to carving.
6. Serve with 1 cup nonstarchy vegetables and ½ cup brown rice.

Cooking tips: Basting the chicken while it cooks will give the chicken an even color and will keep the skin moist. Never cover or tightly wrap a chicken while it is roasting. If a foil cover traps steam, it will cause the chicken to steam rather than roast.

Variation: For Mexican flavor, replace the white wine, mustard, rosemary, and garlic mixture with: 2–3 cloves garlic, chopped; ½ teaspoon ground cumin; 1 teaspoon chopped chipotle in adobo sauce; 1 teaspoon Mexican oregano; and 2 tablespoons lime juice.

Nutrition Facts per Serving of Chicken: calories 320, fat 12 g, carbohydrate 15 g, protein 38 g, sodium 300 mg.

Nutrition Facts per Serving for Mexican Chicken: calories 275, fat 10 g, carbohydrate 8 g, protein 38 g, sodium 600 mg.

Thai Chicken Satay with Peanut Sauce

Start to Finish: 45 minutes, plus 45 minutes for marinating
Stages: 1–7
Yield: 4 servings

FOR SAUCE:

5 dried red chilies
¼ teaspoon ground coriander
¼ teaspoon ground cumin
½ teaspoon kosher or sea salt
1 clove garlic, minced
1 tablespoon minced peeled lemongrass
1 tablespoon minced peeled fresh ginger
1 tablespoon minced shallots or red onion
¾ cup light coconut milk
2 tablespoons creamy all-natural peanut butter
1 tablespoon brown sugar
2 tablespoons fresh lime juice
½ tablespoon fish sauce

FOR CHICKEN:

1 cup light coconut milk
3 tablespoons minced shallots or red onion
2 tablespoons low-sodium soy sauce

1 tablespoon minced peeled fresh ginger
1 teaspoon ground turmeric
1½ pounds chicken breast, trimmed and cut diagonally into thin slices
Cooking spray

1. To prepare chicken: Combine 1 cup coconut milk, shallots, soy sauce, ginger, and turmeric in a large plastic resealable bag.
2. Add chicken to bag, turning to coat. Seal and marinate in refrigerator 45 minutes.
3. To prepare sauce: Place chilies in a small bowl and cover with hot water. Let stand 30 minutes. Drain and finely chop chilies.
4. Combine coriander, cumin, salt, and garlic in small bowl and stir to form a paste. Add chilies, lemongrass, ginger, and shallots, one at a time, until each ingredient is incorporated into the paste.
5. Heat ¾ cup coconut milk in a small saucepan over medium heat. Add paste mixture and cook for 1 minute. Stir in the peanut butter until smooth. Add brown sugar, lime juice, and fish sauce; cook 1 minute. Remove from heat; cool.
6. Remove chicken from bag; discard marinade.
7. Thread chicken slices evenly onto 12 6-inch skewers.
8. Preheat grill or sauté pan, and coat with cooking spray. Place skewers on grill rack or in sauté pan, and cook for 5 minutes on each side or until done.
9. Serve with sauce.

Nutrition Facts per Serving: calories 360, fat 11 g, carbohydrate 22 g, protein 43 g, sodium 900 mg.

Baked Poupon Chicken

Start to Finish: 30 minutes
Stages: 1–7
Yield: 4 servings

4 tablespoons Grey Poupon Dijon Mustard
1½ tablespoons extra-virgin olive oil
1–2 cloves garlic, minced

½ teaspoon Italian seasoning
1⅓ pounds boneless skinless chicken breasts

1. Preheat oven to 375° F.
2. Mix mustard, oil, garlic, and seasoning in a large bowl. Add chicken and turn to coat.
3. Place chicken in baking pan. Bake 20 minutes, or until chicken meat turns white.

Nutrition Facts per Serving: calories 230, fat 8 g, carbohydrate 2 g, protein 36 g, sodium 400 mg.

Spicy Chicken

Start to Finish: 45 minutes
Stages: 1–7
Yield: 4 servings

1⅓ pounds boneless skinless chicken breasts
3 cups low-sodium chicken broth
¼ teaspoon Tabasco sauce
½ teaspoon chili powder
1 tablespoon red pepper flakes
1 teaspoon paprika
1 tablespoon seeded and minced jalapeno pepper (optional)

1. In a large stockpot, combine all ingredients and bring to a boil for 5 minutes.
2. Reduce heat to low, cover, and simmer for 40 minutes.
3. Remove chicken from pot, allow to set 5 minutes to cool, and then shred.

Stage 2 variation: Serve shredded chicken over lettuce and top with salsa.

Stage 3–7 variation: Serve shredded chicken over lettuce and top with salsa and nonfat sour cream.

Nutrition Facts per Serving: calories 180, fat 2.5 g, carbohydrate 2 g, protein 36 g, sodium 377 mg.

Grilled Balsamic Chicken

Start to Finish: 1 hour, plus 4 to 24 hours for marinating
Stages: 1–7
Yield: 6 servings

2 pounds boneless skinless chicken breasts
¼ cup low-sodium chicken broth
½ cup balsamic vinegar
¼ cup chopped scallions
2 tablespoons Dijon mustard
2 cloves garlic, minced
2 teaspoons Worcestershire sauce
1 teaspoon dry mustard
Black pepper to taste

1. Rinse the chicken breasts and pat them dry. Arrange the chicken in a shallow baking dish.
2. In a small bowl, combine the remaining ingredients and whisk to blend well.
3. Pour the marinade over the chicken, cover and refrigerate for at least 12 hours, turning occasionally.
4. Preheat the oven to 325°F. Prepare the grill.
5. Bring chicken and marinade to room temp. Bake in oven for 30 to 40 minutes. Remove the chicken from the marinade and reserve the marinade.
6. Place the chicken on a prepared grill and cook for 5 to 6 minutes on each side, until tender, basting with the reserved marinade.

Nutrition Facts per Serving: calories 190, fat 2.5 g, carbohydrate 6 g, protein 36 g, sodium 245 mg.

Herbed Pork Tenderloin

Start to Finish: 1 hour, plus 2 to 4 hours for marinating
Stages: 1–7
Yield: 8 servings

2 pounds pork tenderloins
Freshly ground black pepper (optional)
2 tablespoons balsamic vinegar
2 tablespoons dry sherry
1 tablespoon cracked black pepper
3 tablespoons extra-virgin olive oil
1 tablespoon soy sauce
2 3-inch sprigs fresh rosemary
2 3-inch sprigs fresh thyme
2 cloves garlic, minced

1. Place meat in a large resealable plastic bag set in a shallow dish. Set aside.
2. For marinade, in a small bowl stir together vinegar, sherry, cracked black pepper, 1 tablespoon of the oil, soy sauce, rosemary, thyme, and garlic. Pour over meat. Seal bag; turn to coat meat. Marinate in the refrigerator for 2 to 4 hours, turning bag occasionally.
3. Preheat oven to 425°F.
4. Drain meat, reserving marinade.
5. In a large skillet heat the remaining 2 tablespoons oil. Brown meat quickly on all sides in hot oil (about 5 minutes).
6. Place meat in a shallow roasting pan. Pour marinade over meat. Insert an oven-safe meat thermometer into the thickest portion of one of the tenderloins. Roast, uncovered, for 15 minutes. Spoon pan juices over meat. Roast for 10 to 15 minutes more or until thermometer registers 155°F. Cover roast with foil and let stand for 15 minutes.
7. The temperature of the meat after standing should be 160°F. Transfer meat to a serving platter, reserving pan juices. Strain juices and pour over meat.

Nutrition Facts per Serving: calories 300, fat 14 g, carbohydrate 2 g, protein 45 g, sodium 100 mg.

Curried Chicken Breasts

Start to Finish: 1 hour 15 minutes, plus 30 minutes for marinating
Stages: 3–7
Yield: 6 servings

½ cup plain nonfat yogurt
3 tablespoons lemon juice
1 tablespoon low-sodium soy sauce
2 teaspoons curry powder
2 pounds boneless skinless chicken breasts

1. In a small bowl, combine yogurt, lemon juice, soy sauce, and curry.
2. Pour over chicken and let sit at room temperature 30 minutes or in refrigerator for several hours.
3. Preheat oven to 375°F.
4. Place marinated chicken in an 8 × 12 baking dish. Bake for 40 minutes or until chicken meat turns white.

Nutrition Facts per Serving: calories 180, fat 2 g, carbohydrate 3 g, protein 36 g, sodium 280 mg.

Tandoori Chicken

Start to Finish: 30 minutes, plus 1 to 3 hours for marinating
Stages: 3–7
Yield: 4 servings

4 boneless skinless chicken breast halves (1 to 1¼ pounds total)
⅛ teaspoon kosher salt
⅛ teaspoon freshly ground black pepper
½ cup plain nonfat Greek yogurt
¼ cup lemon juice
3 cloves garlic, minced
2 teaspoons paprika
¼ teaspoon cayenne pepper
⅛ teaspoon ground cinnamon
⅛ teaspoon ground cumin

1. Sprinkle chicken with kosher salt and black pepper. Place chicken in a resealable plastic bag set in a shallow dish.

2. In a small bowl combine the yogurt, lemon juice, garlic, paprika, cayenne pepper, cinnamon, and cumin. Pour over chicken. Seal bag, turn to coat meat, marinate in the refrigerator for 1 to 3 hours.
3. Remove chicken and discard marinade. For a charcoal grill, place chicken on the rack of an uncovered grill directly over medium coals. Grill for 10 to 12 minutes or until chicken is no longer pink (170°F), turning once halfway through grilling. For a gas grill, preheat grill. Reduce heat to medium. Place chicken on grill rack over heat. Cover and grill as above.

Nutrition Facts per Serving: calories 152, fat 2 g, carbohydrate 5 g, protein 28 g, sodium 144 mg.

Indian-Spiced Pork Loin

Start to Finish: 20 minutes, plus 15 minutes to overnight for marinating
Stages: 3–7
Yield: 4 servings

1 pound pork loin, excess fat removed
1 pinch each salt and pepper
¼ cup plain nonfat Greek yogurt
¼ teaspoon turmeric
¼ teaspoon paprika
½ teaspoon ground cumin
½ teaspoon ground coriander
¼ teaspoon dried mint

1. Season pork with salt and pepper.
2. In a small bowl, combine remaining ingredients and stir to mix. Place in a resealable bag and add pork, forcing out all the air so that the meat is in contact with the marinade. Let sit for 15 minutes to overnight.
3. Preheat grill over medium-high heat. Grill pork until it reaches an internal temperature of 145°F. Allow meat to rest for 10 minutes before slicing.

Variation: Replace pork with 1 pound chicken breast.

Nutrition Facts per Serving: calories 155, fat 4 g, carbohydrate 1.5 g, protein 25 g, sodium 78 mg.

Asian Turkey Meatballs

Start to Finish: 1 hour
Stage: 7
Yield: 4 servings

20 ounces ground turkey (99% fat-free)
¼ cup whole wheat breadcrumbs
1 egg
⅛ teaspoon kosher salt
2 green onions, chopped
1 tablespoon minced fresh ginger
2–3 cloves garlic, minced
¼ cup chopped fresh cilantro
1 tablespoon low-sodium soy sauce
2 teaspoons sesame oil

1. Preheat oven to 400°F.
2. In a bowl, combine and mix ground turkey, breadcrumbs, egg, salt, green onions, ginger, garlic, cilantro, soy sauce, and sesame oil. To avoid excessive dryness, don't overmix or compact the mixture.
3. Divide mixture into 4 ¼-cup portions, shape each portion into a ball, and place on a baking dish. Bake until cooked through, about 15 minutes.

Nutrition Facts per Serving: calories 180, fat 5 g; carbohydrate 4 g, protein 32 g, sodium 550 mg.

Turkey Meatballs

Start to Finish: 30 minutes
Stage: 7
Yield: 6 servings

2 tablespoons extra-virgin olive oil
2 pounds ground turkey breast

1 egg

½ cup whole wheat Italian seasoned breadcrumbs

1. Preheat the oven to 350°F. Grease a 9 × 13 baking dish with the olive oil, and place it in the oven while preheating.
2. In a medium bowl, mix together the ground turkey, egg, and breadcrumbs using your hands.
3. Using an ice cream scoop if possible, form the meat into golf ball–size meatballs. Place about 1 inch apart in the hot baking dish. Press down to flatten the bottom just slightly.
4. Bake for 15 minutes. Then turn them over and continue baking for about 5 more minutes, or until somewhat crispy on the outside.
5. Optional: Serve over 2 cups cooked spaghetti squash or ½ cup cooked whole wheat pasta.

Nutrition Facts per Serving: calories 250, fat 7 g, carbohydrate 7 g, protein 40 g, sodium 232 mg.

Nutrition Facts per Serving with Spaghetti Squash: calories 335, fat 10 g, carbohydrate 27 g, protein 42 g, sodium 266 mg.

Nutrition Facts per Serving with Pasta: calories 285, fat 8 g, carbohydrate 14 g, protein 41 g, sodium 230 mg.

Fish, Seafood, and Tofu Dishes

Mediterranean Grilled Tuna

Start to Finish: 20 minutes
Stages: 1–7
Yield: 4 servings

1 pound fresh or frozen tuna, halibut, or salmon steaks, 1 inch thick

2 teaspoons extra-virgin olive oil

2 teaspoons lemon juice

⅛ teaspoon kosher salt

⅛ teaspoon freshly ground black pepper

2 cloves garlic, minced

2 teaspoons fresh rosemary, or 1 teaspoon dried rosemary or crushed tarragon
1 tablespoon capers, drained and slightly crushed

1. Thaw fish, if frozen. Rinse; pat dry with paper towels. Cut fish into 4 serving-size pieces. Brush both sides with oil and lemon juice; sprinkle with kosher salt and pepper. Sprinkle garlic and rosemary evenly onto fish; rub in with your fingers.
2. For a charcoal grill, place fish on the greased rack of an uncovered grill directly over medium-hot coals. Grill for 8 to 12 minutes or until fish flakes easily when tested with a fork, turning once halfway through grilling. For a gas grill, preheat grill. Reduce heat to medium. Place fish on grill rack over heat. Cover and grill as above.
3. To serve, top fish with capers. If desired, garnish with fresh rosemary.

Broiler method: Place fish on the greased unheated rack of a broiler pan. Broil 4 inches from the heat for 8 to 12 minutes or until fish flakes easily when tested with a fork, turning once halfway through broiling.

Cooking tip: Allow the marinade to sit on the fish for 15 to 30 minutes for the most flavor.

Nutrition Facts per Serving: calories 145, fat 3 g, carbohydrate 1 g, protein 27 g, sodium 179 mg.

Spicy Cod

Start to Finish: 30 minutes
Stages: 1–7
Yield: 3 servings

1 pound cod fillets
1½ tablespoons low-fat mayonnaise
½ teaspoon paprika
½ teaspoon garlic powder
½ teaspoon onion powder
¼ teaspoon pepper

⅛ teaspoon oregano
⅛ teaspoon ground thyme
1 tablespoon lemon juice

1. Preheat oven to 350°F. Thaw fish if frozen.
2. Place thawed or fresh fish fillets on a baking pan.
3. Combine spices and mayonnaise in small bowl. Spread evenly over fish.
4. Bake until fish flakes, approximately 20 to 25 minutes.

Nutrition Facts per Serving: calories 86, fat 1 g, carbohydrate 1 g, protein 17 g, sodium 100 mg.

Sicilian Tuna Steak

Start to Finish: 45 minutes
Stages: 2–7
Yield: 4 servings

1 pound fresh or frozen tuna steaks, 1 inch thick
1 small onion, chopped
2 cloves garlic, minced
1 tablespoon extra-virgin olive oil
2 pounds Roma tomatoes, seeded and chopped, or 1 28-ounce can diced tomatoes, drained
½ cup low-sodium chicken broth
¼ to ½ teaspoon crushed red pepper
¼ cup pitted ripe olives
2 tablespoons capers, rinsed and drained
2 tablespoons chopped fresh basil, or 2 teaspoons crushed dried basil
1 tablespoon chopped fresh mint, or 1 teaspoon crushed dried mint
⅛ teaspoon kosher salt
⅛ teaspoon freshly ground black pepper
1 tablespoon lemon juice

1. Thaw tuna, if frozen. Cut into 4 portions, if necessary. Rinse tuna; pat dry with paper towels. Set aside.
2. In a large skillet, cook onion and garlic in hot oil over medium heat until onion is tender, about 2 minutes. Add tomatoes, broth, and crushed red pepper. Bring to a boil; reduce heat. Simmer, uncovered, for 7 minutes. Add olives, capers, and dried basil and mint, if using; cook for 3 minutes more.
3. Sprinkle tuna with kosher salt and black pepper. Add tuna to skillet on top of tomato mixture. Cover and cook over medium heat for 5 minutes. Uncover and cook for 10 to 15 minutes more or until tuna flakes easily when tested with a fork and is slightly pink in the center.
4. Transfer tuna pieces to 4 serving plates. Spoon tomato mixture over tuna. Sprinkle with fresh basil and mint, if using. Drizzle with lemon juice.

Nutrition Facts per Serving: calories 233, fat 6 g, carbohydrate 12 g, protein 29 g, sodium 377 mg.

Grilled Sesame Salmon Fillet with Scallions

Start to Finish: 30 minutes, plus 30 minutes to 12 hours for marinating
Stages: 1–7
Yield: 4 servings

FOR SALMON:

1¼ pounds salmon fillet, skin on
Vegetable-oil spray or vegetable oil for brushing the grill grate
½ tablespoon toasted sesame seeds
¼ cup thinly sliced scallion greens

FOR MARINADE:

2 tablespoons fresh lime juice
2 tablespoons dry white wine
1 tablespoon low-sodium soy sauce
1 teaspoon Asian sesame oil
1 tablespoon peeled, minced ginger
2 teaspoons minced garlic

⅛ teaspoon red pepper flakes, or ½ teaspoon freshly ground black pepper
¼ cup finely chopped scallions, white parts only

1. To prepare the salmon: Rinse, pat dry, and remove any bones, if needed. Place salmon skin-side down in a nonreactive pan or on a platter with a lip.
2. To prepare the marinade: Combine all ingredients in a bowl; mix well. Pour mixture over the salmon and then turn the salmon skin-side up. Cover the pan or platter with plastic wrap and place the fish in the refrigerator for at least 30 minutes and up to 12 hours.
3. Preheat the grill.
4. When the grill is hot, remove the grill grate, and spray or brush the grate with the vegetable oil, then replace the grate on the grill. When you are sure the grate is hot, place fish on it, skin-side up.
5. Grill the fish for about 5 minutes, then turn it and grill about 5 minutes longer for a total of 10 minutes. When the fish is done, remove it to a serving platter skin-side down and sprinkle the fish with the sesame seeds and scallion greens.

Nutrition Facts per Serving: calories 260, fat 15 g, carbohydrate 1 g, protein 29 g, sodium 350 mg.

Grilled Salmon with Mustard Sauce

Start to Finish: 30 minutes
Stages: 1–7
Yield: 4 servings

FOR SALMON:

4 salmon fillets, about 6 ounces each
1 lemon, halved
freshly ground black pepper

FOR SAUCE:

½ cup Dijon mustard
1 teaspoon extra-virgin olive oil

1–2 cloves garlic, minced
1 tablespoon dried dill
1 handful chopped fresh basil

1. To prepare salmon: Rinse fillets and pat dry. Squeeze juice from half of the lemon over the fillets; season them with pepper. Preheat grill or broiler.
2. To prepare the sauce: Whisk together mustard, olive oil, garlic, and dill in a small bowl. Add basil and juice from the other half of the lemon; mix well.
3. Grill the fish on high heat or broil for approximately 10 to 15 minutes, being careful not to overcook.
4. Spoon sauce over the fish and serve immediately.

Nutrition Facts per Serving: calories 360, fat 22 g, carbohydrate 4 g, protein 36 g, sodium 680 mg.

Ginger Lime Fish

Start to Finish: 30 minutes, plus 30 minutes for marinating
Stages: 1–7
Yield: 4 servings

1⅓ pounds thick fish fillets such as cod or halibut
2 teaspoons finely grated fresh ginger
1 tablespoon low-sodium soy sauce
¼ cup lime juice

1. Preheat oven to 375°F. Place the fillet skin-side down in a baking dish coated with nonstick spray.
2. Combine the ginger, soy sauce, and lime juice. Pour over the fish and marinate for at least 30 minutes.
3. Bake for 20 to 25 minutes, or until the fish is opaque.

Nutrition Facts per Serving with Cod: calories 130, fat 1 g, carbohydrate 2 g, protein 27 g, sodium 300 mg.

Nutrition Facts per Serving with Halibut: calories 170, fat 3.5 g, carbohydrate 2 g, protein 32 g, sodium 300 mg.

Crustless Smoked Salmon Quiche with Dill

Start to Finish: 45 minutes
Stages: 5–7
Yield: 2 servings

1¼ cups nonfat evaporated milk
¼ cup nonfat sour cream
1 teaspoon Dijon mustard
4 large egg whites
1 large egg
½ cup (2 ounces) shredded Cabot Sharp Light cheese
½ cup thinly sliced green onions
¼ cup chopped smoked salmon
2 tablespoons chopped fresh dill
½ teaspoon freshly ground black pepper
Cooking spray

1. Preheat oven to 350°F.
2. Combine evaporated milk, sour cream, mustard, egg whites, and egg in a large bowl and whisk. Stir in cheese, onions, salmon, dill, and pepper.
3. Pour egg mixture into 9-inch pie plate coated with cooking spray.
4. Bake for 35 minutes. Let stand 15 minutes. Serve warm from the oven or chilled.

Nutrition Facts per Serving: calories 340, fat 9 g, carbohydrate 28 g, protein 36 g, sodium 900 mg.

Fish Poached in Spicy Chipotle Broth

Start to Finish: 30 minutes
Stages: 6–7
Yield: 4 servings

1 tablespoon extra-virgin olive oil
1 cup sliced onions
2 cloves garlic, chopped
1 teaspoon chopped chipotle chilies in adobo sauce

Pinch of cumin seeds
1 cup canned low-sodium tomatoes, drained, chopped
1½ cups low-sodium chicken broth
1 cup garbanzo beans, drained; reserve ¼ cup liquid
Salt and pepper to taste
1 tablespoon chopped cilantro or parsley (optional)
1 cup spinach (optional)
2 pounds fish such as salmon, cod, halibut, or sea bass

1. Heat a large sauté pan over medium heat. Add olive oil and onions; sauté for 4 minutes or until slightly caramelized. Add garlic, chipotle, and cumin seeds; cook 15 seconds. Add tomatoes, chicken broth, garbanzo beans and their liquid. Bring to a simmer. Cook for 10 minutes or until the flavors have melded. Season with salt and pepper. Add optional herbs and spinach; cook to wilt, 1 to 2 minutes.
2. Add fish in a single layer. Cover and simmer for 5 to 6 minutes or until fish flakes easily when tested with a fork.
3. Using a slotted spatula, carefully transfer fish to a platter. Serve with sauce and vegetables.

Cooking tips: Make this broth ahead without the herbs and spinach. It will freeze well. You can also use this as a sauce for chicken or eggs.

Variations: For Spanish flavor, replace the chipotle chilies with 1 teaspoon Spanish paprika. Add ¼ cup roasted red peppers when the tomatoes are added. Or for a Mediterranean dish, replace the chipotle chilies, cumin seeds, and garbanzo beans with white beans and basil. Serve with basil pesto on top.

Nutrition Facts per Serving: calories 310, fat 7 g, carbohydrate 25 g, protein 40 g, sodium 300 mg.

Glazed Salmon with Avocado Slaw*

Start to Finish: 25 minutes
Stages: 2-7
Yield: 4 servings

3 tablespoons soy sauce
1 clove garlic, peeled
1 teaspoon peeled and finely chopped fresh ginger
2½ tablespoons honey
1 teaspoon sesame oil
¼ cup seasoned rice vinegar
¼ cup olive oil
4 (5 oz.) salmon filets
¼ cup sliced water chestnuts, cut into thin strips
1 medium carrot, shredded
1 red bell pepper, thinly sliced
3 cups shredded Napa cabbage
Salt and ground black pepper, to taste
1 large, ripe Fresh California Avocado, peeled, seeded, and cut into ¼-inch cubes

1. Place soy sauce, garlic, ginger, honey, sesame oil, vinegar and olive oil in a food processor or blender. Blend until smooth and creamy.
2. Place salmon filets in a shallow dish and pour half the soy sauce mixture over top; turn filets to coat on all sides. Set aside.
3. Place water chestnuts, carrot, bell pepper and cabbage in a medium bowl and toss with remaining soy sauce mixture. Season with salt and pepper. Add avocado and toss to combine. Set aside.
4. Heat small amount of olive oil in a non-stick skillet over medium high heat. Place salmon skin-side up and cook until nicely browned, about 6 minutes. Turn salmon over and cook until it is cooked through, about 6 minutes more.
5. Plate salmon and spoon slaw over each filet.

Cooking tip: Large avocados are recommended for this recipe. A large avocado averages about 8 ounces. If using smaller or larger size avoca-

---

* Recipe provided by California Avocado Commission. Copyright © 2015

dos adjust the quantity accordingly. As with all fruits and vegetables, wash avocados before cutting.

Nutrition Information Per Serving: calories 390, fat 17 g, carbohydrate 26 g; protein 32 g; sodium 380 mg.

Shrimp Avocado Stir-Fry*

Start to Finish: 20 minutes
Stages: 2-7
Yield: 4 servings

Cooking spray, as needed
1 cup baby carrots
1 red bell pepper, cored, seeded, sliced in thin strips
1 package of fresh stir-fry vegetables with broccoli
1 pound cooked large shrimp
⅓ cup low-sodium teriyaki sauce**
1 large, ripe Fresh California Avocado, peeled, seeded, and diced

1. Coat large nonstick skillet or wok with cooking spray and place over medium-high heat.
2. Add carrots, bell pepper, and package of vegetables to skillet.
3. Cook, stirring constantly, until all vegetables are crisp-tender, about 5 minutes.
4. Add shrimp and teriyaki sauce, stir to heat through.
5. Evenly distribute onto four serving plates, and top with equal portions of diced avocado.

Cooking tip: Large avocados are recommended for this recipe. A large avocado averages about 8 ounces. If using smaller or larger size avocados adjust the quantity accordingly. As with all fruits and vegetables, wash avocados before cutting.

Nutrition Information Per Serving: calories 252, fat 8 g, carbohydrate 20 g; protein 27 g; sodium 845 mg.

---

* Recipe provided by California Avocado Commission. Copyright © 2015

** Look for a low-sodium teriyaki sauce that has less than 5 grams of sugar. Kikkoman Less Sodium Teriyaki Marinade & Sauce is one option.

Curried Tofu

Start to Finish: 30 minutes
Stages: 1–7
Yield: 4 servings

FOR SAUCE:

1 cup light coconut milk
2 tablespoons chopped fresh cilantro
1 teaspoon red curry paste
½ teaspoon brown sugar
½ teaspoon kosher salt

FOR TOFU AND VEGETABLES:

2 12-ounce packages extra-firm low-fat or light tofu
Cooking spray
4 cups baby spinach
1 medium red bell pepper, sliced

1. To prepare sauce: Whisk all ingredients together in a small bowl.
2. To prepare tofu and vegetables: Drain, rinse, and pat dry tofu. Slice block crosswise into 8-inch slabs. Coarsely crumble each slice into bite-size pieces.
3. Heat large nonstick skillet over medium-high heat, coat with cooking spray, and add tofu pieces in a single layer. Once tofu has browned (about 5 minutes), gently stir and continue cooking, stirring occasionally, until all sides are golden brown. Add spinach, bell pepper, and curry sauce and cook until heated through, 1 to 2 minutes.

Nutrition Facts per Serving: calories 269, fat 14 g, carbohydrate 15 g, protein 20 g, sodium 475 mg.

Breakfast Dishes

Baked Eggs with Grilled Vegetables

Start to Finish: 25 minutes
Stages: 3–7
Yield: 4 servings

1 teaspoon extra-virgin olive oil
1 clove garlic, minced
1 tablespoon basil, chopped
¼ cup (1 ounce) low-fat mozzarella cheese, cut into ¼-inch pieces
4 cups grilled vegetables, cut into ½-inch pieces
4 slices tomato
6 eggs
1 tablespoon grated Parmesan cheese
Salt and pepper to taste

1. Preheat oven to 325°F.
2. Lightly oil 4 4-inch-diameter ovenproof glass or ceramic dishes with olive oil.
3. In a bowl, mix together the garlic, basil, mozzarella cheese, and grilled vegetables; season with salt and pepper.
4. Place 1 slice of tomato in bottom of each baking dish. Divide vegetable mixture among the 4 dishes. Crack an egg into each dish. Season with salt and pepper. Sprinkle with Parmesan cheese.
5. Bake for 10 to 15 minutes or until the vegetables are warm and the egg whites are cooked through.
6. Serve immediately.

Nutrition Facts per Serving: calories 130, fat 7 g, carbohydrate 9 g, protein 12 g, sodium 139 mg.

Variations: Replace grilled vegetables with roasted vegetables or leftover sautéed spinach and mushrooms. Replace mozzarella cheese with feta cheese.

Avocado, Fruit, and Citrus Bowl*

Start to Finish: 10 minutes
Stages: 4-7
Yield: 2 servings

2 teaspoons grated orange peel
2 teaspoons grated lemon peel
¼ cup fresh lemon juice
1 tablespoon sugar
1 cup cantaloupe balls or ¾ inch cubes
1 cup honeydew balls or ¾ inch cubes
1 large, ripe Fresh California Avocado, peeled, seeded, and cut into chunks
1 cup orange sections, cut in half
½ cup fresh raspberries

1. Combine orange peel, lemon peel, lemon juice, and sugar in a small bowl. Stir until well blended.
2. Spoon half of the melon balls, avocado, orange sections, and raspberries in a shallow pan, such as a 1½-qt casserole dish. Repeat layers. Do not toss. Drizzle citrus mixture evenly over all.

Cooking Tip: Large avocados are recommended for this recipe. A large avocado averages about 8 ounces. If using smaller or larger size avocados adjust the quantity accordingly. As with all fruits and vegetables, wash avocados before cutting.

Nutrition Information Per Serving: calories 160, fat 9 g, carbohydrate 23 g; protein 2 g; sodium 20 mg.

Anytime Omelet*

Start to Finish: 15 minutes
Stages: 5-7
Yield: 2 servings

3 eggs, lightly beaten
3 tablespoons low-fat milk

---

* Recipe provided by California Avocado Commission. Copyright © 2015

Nonstick cooking spray
½ cup shredded low-fat cheddar cheese
1 tablespoon sliced green onion
¼ cup chopped red bell pepper
1 large, ripe Fresh California Avocado, peeled, seeded, and cubed

1. Mix eggs and milk.
2. Spray a large skillet with nonstick cooking spray and heat over medium low heat. Pour egg mixture into skillet. Cook eggs until top is almost set.
3. Sprinkle with cheese and green onion. Cook until cheese melts, about 2 minutes.
4. Top with red pepper and avocado, fold over and serve immediately.

Cooking Tip: Large avocados are recommended for this recipe. A large avocado averages about 8 ounces. If using smaller or larger size avocados adjust the quantity accordingly. As with all fruits and vegetables, wash avocados before cutting.

Nutrition Information Per Serving: calories 310, fat 23 g, carbohydrate 11 g; protein 16 g; sodium 210 mg.

Roasted Vegetables

The nutritional information here applies to the recipes for Asparagus and Mushrooms, Carrots, Cauliflower, Broccoli, Cabbage, and Roasted Brussels Sprouts. Be sure to give each a try, and don't be afraid of creating different combinations until you find your favorite roasted veggie blend.

Start to Finish: 20 to 35 minutes
Stages: 2–7
Yield: 4 servings

Nutrition Facts per Serving (approximate for each vegetable): calories 50, carbohydrate 7 g, fat 2 g, protein 1 g, sodium 100 mg.

Zucchini

2 cloves garlic, minced
1 tablespoon extra-virgin olive oil
1 teaspoon dry oregano
½ teaspoon freshly ground black pepper
¼ teaspoon kosher salt
1½ pounds (about 6 cups) zucchini and/or yellow summer squash, sliced ½-inch thick

1. Preheat oven to 425°F.
2. In a small saucepan, heat oil over medium heat and cook garlic for 30 seconds. Stir in oregano, pepper, and kosher salt.
3. Place zucchini in a 13 × 9 × 2 baking pan; add oil mixture. Toss to coat.
4. Roast, uncovered, for about 20 minutes or until crisp-tender, stirring once.

Nutrition Facts per Serving: calories 61, fat 4 g, carbohydrate 6 g, protein 2 g, sodium 138 mg.

Asparagus and Mushrooms

1 cup raw mushrooms
1 cup asparagus
1 tablespoon oil

1. Preheat oven to 400°F.
2. Roll asparagus and/or whole small mushrooms around on an oiled tray until they are lightly coated.
3. Roast for only 5 to 10 minutes, or until just tender.
4. Salt lightly while still hot, and serve at any temperature.

Carrots

2 cups carrots
1 tablespoon oil

1. Preheat oven to 375°F.
2. Cut larger carrots into 2-inch lengths; leave small ones whole.
3. Roll the vegetables around on an oiled baking tray until they are lightly coated.
4. Roast for 30 minutes or until done to your liking.
5. Serve at any temperature.

Cauliflower

2 cups cauliflower
1 tablespoon oil

1. Preheat oven to 375°F.
2. Break cauliflower into 1½-inch florets, place on an oiled tray, and roll around until they are lightly coated.
3. Roast for 15 minutes.
4. Salt lightly while still hot, and serve at any temperature.

Broccoli

2 cups broccoli florets
1 tablespoon oil

1. Preheat oven to 400°F.
2. Peel broccoli stems and cut off from the base of the crown. Cut stems and crown into 2-inch chunks.
3. Place in an oiled baking dish and roast for 20 to 25 minutes, depending on the thickness of the pieces.

Cabbage

2 cups cabbage, cut into 2-inch wedges
1 tablespoon oil

1. Preheat oven to 400°F.
2. Toss cabbage in oil, making sure all pieces are well covered.
3. Roast for about 20 minutes.

Brussels Sprouts

2 cups Brussels sprouts
1 tablespoon oil

1. Preheat oven to 400°F.
2. Cut large Brussels sprouts in half and leave smaller ones whole, making sure they are as uniform in size as possible.
3. Toss in oil, making sure all pieces are well covered.
4. Roast for 15 to 20 minutes, depending on the size.

Side Dishes, Dips, Sauces, and Snacks

Steamed Spaghetti Squash

Start to Finish: 1 hour
Stages: 2–7
Yield: 4 servings

1 spaghetti squash (3 pounds)
Salt and pepper to taste
Water

1. Preheat oven to 400°F.
2. Cut squash in half; scoop out seeds with a spoon. Season with salt and pepper. Place 2 tablespoons water in the cavity of each half.
3. Place in a baking dish and add ½ cup water to the bottom of the pan. Cover tightly with foil and bake in the oven for 40 to 50 minutes or until the squash is soft enough to pull the flesh from the

skin in strands. The squash may still be a bit crunchy, but it should pull easily from the skin.

4. Gently pull at the flesh with a fork to separate it into spaghetti strands. Season with salt and pepper.

Cooking tip: When pulling the squash from the skin, you may have to do it in sections. Pull the top portion of the flesh, and then place the squash back in the oven to cook a little more. The squash should be a little crunchy, not soft and mushy. Can be served hot as a side vegetable or cold as a salad.

Variations: Sprinkle with 3 tablespoons lemon juice, 1 tablespoon extra-virgin olive oil, and 1 tablespoon each chopped basil and parsley. Or you can add 2 tablespoons capers, 1 tablespoon chopped oregano, 1 cup chopped tomatoes, 1 teaspoon extra-virgin olive oil, and 3 tablespoons red wine vinegar.

Nutrition Facts per Serving: calories 100, fat 2 g, carbohydrate 23 g, protein 2 g, sodium 55 mg.

Coconut Lime Cauliflower "Rice"

Start to Finish: 30 minutes
Stages: 2–7
Yield: 4 servings

1 large head cauliflower (stems and leaves removed), separated into pieces
1 tablespoon extra-virgin olive oil
½ cup chopped fresh cilantro
Juice of ½ lime
1 tablespoon minced garlic
2 tablespoons canned light coconut milk
⅛ teaspoon kosher salt

1. Rinse cauliflower and dry well with paper towels. Next, "rice" your cauliflower by either pulsing it in a food processor, taking care not to over-process into a purée, or grating it with a fine cheese grater.

2. Heat oil in a large saucepan over medium heat, and then add in cauliflower "rice," cilantro, lime juice, and garlic.
3. Cook until cauliflower is hot throughout; then add coconut milk and salt. Cook for an additional 2 minutes and serve warm.

Nutrition Facts per Serving: calories 74, fat 3 g, carbohydrate 8.5 g, protein 3 g, sodium 200 mg.

Garlic Sautéed Greens

Start to Finish: 20 minutes
Stages: 2–7
Yield: 4 servings

8 cups chopped raw greens
1 tablespoon extra-virgin olive oil
2 cloves garlic, minced
1 teaspoon lemon juice
½ teaspoon tamari or low-sodium soy sauce

1. Wash greens carefully (for greens with tough stems, cut the leaves away from the stem before washing). An easy way to do this is to fill your sink with cold water and submerge the greens. If the water has a lot of sediment, drain the sink and repeat. Drain greens and chop.
2. Heat oil in a 10-inch skillet. Add garlic and sauté a minute or so. Add greens and keep them moving in the skillet, turning frequently so that all the greens reach the heat.
3. When all greens have turned bright green and begun to wilt, remove from heat. Sprinkle lemon juice and tamari or soy sauce over the top.
4. Toss gently and serve.

Nutrition Facts per Serving: calories 70, fat 4 g, carbohydrate 5 g, protein 2 g, sodium 45 mg.

Savory Asparagus

Start to Finish: 20 minutes
Stages: 2–7
Yield: 4 servings

1½ pounds asparagus, ends snapped off
1 tablespoon low-sodium soy sauce
1 teaspoon dark sesame oil
2 drops chili oil
½ teaspoon sesame seeds

1. Cut asparagus slightly diagonally into pieces 2 inches long.
2. Bring a pot of water to a boil. Add asparagus and cook 1½ to 2 minutes. Drain and place asparagus in an ice bath for 3 minutes. Drain again, then pat dry completely.
3. In a bowl, combine soy sauce, oils, and asparagus. Toss to combine; then toss with sesame seeds and serve.

Nutrition Facts per Serving: calories 50, carbohydrate 7 g, fat 2 g, protein 1 g, sodium 150 mg.

Red Pepper Hummus

Start to Finish: 30 minutes
Stages: 6–7
Yield: 8 servings

1 red bell pepper
2½ tablespoons fresh lemon juice
1 tablespoon tahini
¼ teaspoon freshly ground black pepper
½ teaspoon kosher salt
¼ teaspoon ground cumin
1 15-ounce can garbanzo beans, rinsed and drained
1 garlic clove, minced

1. Preheat broiler.
2. Halve bell pepper lengthwise and discard seeds and membranes. Place pepper halves, skin side up, on foil-lined baking sheet and flatten with hand. Broil 10 minutes or until blackened.

3. Let cool. Close in a resealable plastic bag, let stand 10 minutes, and then peel skins.
4. Combine bell pepper with remaining ingredients in food processor and process until smooth.
5. Serve with crackers or sliced veggies for dipping.

Nutrition Facts per Serving: calories 60, fat 2 g, carbohydrate 9 g, protein 3 g, sodium 325 mg.

Cucumber Raita

Start to Finish: 15 minutes
Stages: 3-7
Yield: 2 servings

2 cups plain nonfat Greek yogurt
1 teaspoon roasted cumin powder
Chili powder and ground pepper to taste (optional)
1 cucumber, chopped
Few sprigs of cilantro, chopped
1 serving healthy fat
½ cup sliced vegetables (carrots, celery, cucumbers), for dipping

1. Stir together yogurt, cumin, and chili powder or pepper, if using; mix until smooth. Add chopped cucumber and chopped cilantro to mixture.
2. Mix 1 serving of healthy fat—10 olives; 1 tablespoon sunflower seeds, pumpkin seeds, or sesame seeds; or 6 almonds—into cucumber raita.
3. Enjoy with vegetables of your choice.

Nutrition Facts per Serving: calories 137, fat 5 g, carbohydrate 9 g, protein 14 g, sodium 120 mg.

Cilantro Mint Sauce

Start to Finish: 15 minutes
Stages: 1–7
Yield: 6 servings

1 bunch cilantro leaves
1 bunch mint leaves
½ cup pine nuts
¼ cup champagne vinegar
2 cloves garlic, chopped
Juice of 2 limes
½ teaspoon ground cumin
½ teaspoon red pepper
½ cup broth

1. Place all ingredients in a food processor and puree until consistency is creamy.
2. Drizzle on skewers, grilled meats, seafood, or soups, or serve on the side.

Nutrition Facts per Serving: calories 50, fat 3 g, carbohydrate 6 g, protein 2 g, sodium 110 mg.

Cheese Crisps

Start to Finish: 15 minutes
Stages: 3–7
Yield: 2 servings

2 ounces low-fat cheese (dry varieties)
Cayenne pepper to taste
Garlic powder to taste

1. Preheat oven to 350°F.
2. Cut low-fat cheese into squares and place onto cooking sheet. Sprinkle with cayenne pepper and garlic powder to taste. Bake for approximately 7 minutes.

Nutrition Facts per Serving: calories 70, fat 4.5 g, carbohydrate 1 g, protein 9 g, sodium 200 mg.

CHAPTER 16

The Love Diet Meal Plans

One of the challenges in starting a new eating plan is knowing how to eat throughout the day. In this chapter, we've included sample menus for men and women for three days during each stage—this will help you begin to develop a sense of how to plan your meals and snacks. Use these as templates to get you started and then be sure to branch off and add in different recipes and foods as you grow more confident with the program.

Stage 1: Women

1,100–1,400 calories per day

Day 1

BREAKFAST

1 cup egg whites scrambled with cooking spray, topped with a dash of paprika and black pepper for a quick and easy flavor boost

1 cup berries

1 tablespoon nut butter

LUNCH

4 ounces Avocado Tuna Salad (page 211)

1 cup mixed berries

SNACK

2 ounces cooked chicken breast, no skin

1 cup berries

DINNER

6 ounces fish in Asian Herb Marinade (page 195)

1 cup berries

Day 2

BREAKFAST

20/20 LifeStyles High Protein Shake

1 tablespoon nut butter

1 cup blueberries

LUNCH

4 ounces grilled chicken breast prepared with a favorite marinade or spice rub from Chapter 14

⅛ avocado

1 cup berries

SNACK

2 hard-boiled eggs

1 cup berries

DINNER

6 ounces Grilled Salmon with Mustard Sauce (page 244)

1 cup berries

Day 3

BREAKFAST

1 cup egg whites scrambled with canola or olive oil spray

1 tablespoon nut butter

1 cup berries

LUNCH

4 ounces cooked very lean ground beef (5% fat), prepared with your favorite fresh herb and spice seasonings

6 almonds, chopped and added to 1 cup strawberries

SNACK

20/20 LifeStyles Protein Bar

DINNER

6 ounces pork tenderloin marinated in Chipotle Lime Marinade (page 197) and grilled

1 cup berries

Stage 1: Men

1,300–1,700 calories per day

Day 1

BREAKFAST

1 cup egg whites scrambled with cooking spray, topped with a dash of paprika and black pepper for a quick and easy flavor boost

1 cup strawberries

1 tablespoon nut butter

SNACK

2 ounces sliced low-sodium turkey breast

1 cup raspberries

LUNCH

6 ounces Avocado Tuna Salad (page 211)

1 cup berries

SNACK

2 ounces cooked chicken breast, no skin

1 cup berries

DINNER

8 ounces fish marinated in Asian Herb Marinade (page 195)

1 cup berries

Day 2

BREAKFAST

20/20 LifeStyles High Protein Shake

1 tablespoon nut butter

1 cup strawberries

SNACK

2 hard-boiled eggs

1 cup blueberries

LUNCH

6 ounces grilled chicken breast flavored with lemon or lime, herbs, or a flavorful marinade or rub from Chapter 14

⅛ avocado

1 cup berries

SNACK

2 ounces grilled chicken breast

1 cup berries

DINNER

8 ounces Grilled Salmon with Mustard Sauce (page 244)

1 cup berries

Day 3

BREAKFAST

1 cup egg whites scrambled in 1 teaspoon extra-virgin olive oil or canola oil, or 2 whole eggs scrambled with no added oil

1 tablespoon nut butter

1 cup berries

SNACK

2 ounces sliced low-sodium turkey breast

1 cup berries

LUNCH

6 ounces cooked very lean ground beef (5% fat), prepared with your favorite fresh herb and spice seasonings

6 almonds, chopped and added to 1 cup strawberries

SNACK

20/20 LifeStyles Protein Bar

DINNER

8 ounces pork tenderloin marinated in Chipotle Lime Marinade (page 197) and grilled

1 cup berries

Stage 2: Women

1,100–1,400 calories per day

Day 1

BREAKFAST

Veggie omelet: 1 cup egg whites, ½ cup chopped bell peppers, ¼ cup chopped tomatoes, and 1 teaspoon oil

1 cup strawberries

LUNCH

4 ounces grilled chicken breast prepared with Chermoula Marinade (page 196) and grilled

Green salad: 1½ cups salad greens (any lettuce but iceberg), ¼ cup chopped carrots, ¼ cup chopped tomatoes, 2 tablespoons low-fat salad dressing such as 1 teaspoon extra-virgin olive oil with choice of vinegar (see pages 208–211 for more options)

1 cup berries

SNACK

2 ounces sliced low-sodium turkey breast

1 cup blueberries

DINNER

6 ounces Turkey Meatballs (page 239) with 1½ cups Steamed Spaghetti Squash (page 256)

1 cup berries

Day 2

BREAKFAST

Turkey sausage egg scramble: ½ cup egg whites, 2 ounces lean turkey sausage, 1 teaspoon olive oil

1 cup berries

LUNCH

4 ounces Grilled Balsamic Chicken (page 235)

6 almonds

1 cup steamed broccoli with ½ cup tomatoes

1 cup strawberries

SNACK

1 cup berries

½ cup shelled edamame

DINNER

6 ounces flank steak prepared with Spanish Marinade (page 198) and grilled

1½ cups grilled asparagus

1 cup berries

Day 3

BREAKFAST

20/20 LifeStyles High Protein Shake made with 1 tablespoon nut butter and 1 cup berries

LUNCH

4 ounces shrimp marinated with Asian Herb Marinade (page 195) and grilled, served over 1½ cups salad greens mixed with ½ cup asparagus, ½ cup marinated artichoke hearts, and 1 teaspoon Simple Lemon Vinaigrette (page 209)

1 cup berries

SNACK

2 ounces low-sodium sliced turkey breast

1 cup berries

DINNER

6 ounces pork tenderloin prepared with Jamaican Jerk Rub (page 200) and grilled

1½ cups Roasted Brussels Sprouts (page 256)

1 cup berries

Stage 2: Men

1,300–1,700 calories per day

Day 1

BREAKFAST

Veggie omelet: 1 cup egg whites, ½ cup chopped bell peppers, ¼ cup chopped tomatoes, and 1 teaspoon oil

1 cup strawberries

1 tablespoon nut butter

SNACK

20/20 LifeStyles Protein Bar

LUNCH

6 ounces grilled chicken breast marinated in Chermoula Marinade (page 196)

Green salad: 1½ cups salad greens, ¼ cup chopped carrots, ¼ cup chopped tomatoes, and 2 tablespoons low-fat salad dressing such as 1 teaspoon extra-virgin olive oil with choice of vinegar

1 cup berries

SNACK

2 ounces sliced low-sodium turkey breast

1 cup blueberries

DINNER

8 ounces Turkey Meatballs (page 239) with 1½ cups Steamed Spaghetti Squash (page 256)

1 cup berries

Day 2

BREAKFAST

Turkey sausage egg scramble: ½ cup egg whites, 2 ounces lean turkey sausage, 1 teaspoon olive oil

1 cup raspberries

LUNCH

6 ounces Grilled Balsamic Chicken (page 235)

6 almonds

1 cup steamed broccoli with ½ cup tomatoes

1 cup strawberries

SNACK

1 cup berries

½ cup shelled edamame

DINNER

8 ounces flank steak marinated in Spanish Marinade (page 198) and grilled

1½ cups grilled asparagus

1 cup berries

Day 3

BREAKFAST

20/20 LifeStyles High Protein Shake with 1 tablespoon nut butter and 1 cup berries

SNACK

2 ounces low-sodium turkey breast

1 cup berries

LUNCH

6 ounces salmon marinated in Asian Herb Marinade (page 195) and grilled, served over 1½ cups greens with 1 cup mixed asparagus and artichoke hearts

1 cup berries

SNACK

½ cup shelled edamame

1 cup berries

DINNER

8 ounces pork tenderloin prepared with Jamaican Jerk Rub (page 200), grilled or roasted

1½ cups steamed green beans

1 cup berries

Stage 3: Women

1,100–1,400 calories per day

Day 1

BREAKFAST

1 cup plain nonfat Greek yogurt
1 cup raspberries
12 almonds

LUNCH

4 ounces chicken breast prepared with Fresh Herb Rub (page 199) and grilled
Spinach salad: 1½ cups spinach, 1 cup mixed raw veggies, 2 tablespoons low-calorie dressing of your choice (page 208)
1 cup berries

SNACK

2 ounces low-sodium turkey breast
1 cup strawberries

DINNER

6 ounces pork tenderloin marinated in Chipotle Lime Marinade (page 197) and grilled
1½ cups steamed green beans
1 cup berries

Day 2

BREAKFAST

Canadian bacon scramble: ½ cup egg whites scrambled with canola or olive oil spray, 1 ounce low-sodium Canadian bacon, ¼ cup (1 ounce) shredded low-fat Cheddar cheese
⅛ avocado
1 cup strawberries

LUNCH

Stuffed peppers with ground-beef-and-vegetable medley: Halve and seed two small green bell peppers and set aside; add 1 teaspoon olive oil to a skillet and brown 4 ounces lean ground beef (5% fat) with ½ onion, chopped. Add ½ cup jarred marinara sauce to browned meat and heat for an additional 5 minutes. Fill the peppers with the ground beef and serve.

1 cup blueberries

SNACK

2 ounces low-sodium turkey jerky, deli meat, or cooked chicken

1 cup blueberries

DINNER

6 ounces salmon marinated in Asian Herb Marinade (page 195) and grilled

1½ cups Grilled Asparagus Salad (page 214)

1 cup berries

Day 3

BREAKFAST

1 cup nonfat plain Greek yogurt

1 cup berries

12 almonds

LUNCH

Chicken Caesar salad: 4 ounces grilled chicken breast, 1½ cups romaine lettuce, ½ cup sliced cucumber, 2 tablespoons light Caesar dressing

1 cup berries

SNACK

20/20 LifeStyles Protein Bar

DINNER

6 ounces lean beef such as filet mignon or sirloin, grilled

1 cup steamed zucchini and yellow squash

1½ cups mixed green salad

1 tablespoon salad dressing

1 cup berries

Stage 3: Men

1,300–1,700 calories per day

Day 1

BREAKFAST

1 cup nonfat plain Greek Yogurt
1 cup raspberries
12 almonds

SNACK

20/20 LifeStyles Protein Bar

LUNCH

6 ounces chicken prepared with Fresh Herb Rub (page 199) and grilled
Spinach salad: 1½ cups spinach, 1 cup mixed raw veggies, and 2 tablespoons choice of low-calorie dressing
1 cup berries

SNACK

2 ounces lean turkey breast
1 cup strawberries

DINNER

8 ounces pork tenderloin marinated in Chipotle Lime Marinade (page 197) and grilled
1½ cups steamed green beans
1 cup berries

Day 2

BREAKFAST

Canadian bacon scramble: 1½ cups egg whites scrambled in 1 teaspoon olive oil with 1 ounce low-sodium Canadian bacon and ¼ cup (1 ounce) shredded low-fat Cheddar cheese
⅛ avocado
1 cup strawberries

LUNCH

Stuffed peppers with ground-beef-and-vegetable-medley: Halve and seed two small green bell peppers and set aside; add 1 teaspoon olive oil to a skillet and brown 6 ounces lean ground beef with ½ onion, chopped. Add ½ cup jarred marinara sauce to browned meat and heat for an additional 5 minutes. Fill the peppers with the ground beef and serve.

1 cup blueberries

SNACK

2 ounces low-sodium turkey jerky, deli meat, or cooked chicken

1 cup blueberries

DINNER

8 ounces salmon marinated in Asian Herb Marinade (page 195)

1½ cups grilled asparagus with 1 teaspoon olive oil

1 cup berries

Day 3

BREAKFAST

1 cup nonfat plain Greek yogurt

1 cup berries

12 almonds

SNACK

2 ounces low-sodium turkey deli meat

1 cup berries

LUNCH

Chicken Caesar salad: 6 ounces grilled chicken breast, 1½ cups romaine lettuce, ½ cup sliced cucumber, 2 tablespoons light Caesar dressing

1 cup berries

SNACK

20/20 LifeStyles Protein Bar, or 1 low-fat string cheese with 1 cup berries

DINNER

8 ounces lean beef such as filet mignon or sirloin, grilled

1 cup steamed zucchini and yellow squash

1½ cups mixed green salad, with 1 tablespoon dressing (see page 208 for dressing options)

1 cup berries

Stage 4: Women

1,100–1,400 calories per day

Day 1

BREAKFAST

2 ounces turkey sausage

½ cup low-fat cottage cheese mixed with ¼ cup raspberries, ½ cup blueberries, and 10 walnut halves

LUNCH

4 ounces salmon prepared with Mustard-Peppercorn Rub (page 200) and grilled

Steamed-vegetable medley: ½ cup cauliflower, ½ cup broccoli, and ½ cup carrots

1 medium apple (tennis ball size)

SNACK

20/20 LifeStyles Protein Bar or 2 ounces low-sodium sliced turkey breast and 1 cup berries

DINNER

4 ounces Roast Chicken (page 231)

Spinach salad: 1½ cups spinach leaves, ¼ cup sliced radishes, ¼ cup chopped tomatoes, 1 tablespoon dressing of your choice (page 208)

½ cup grapes

Day 2

BREAKFAST

1 cup egg whites scrambled with 1 teaspoon extra-virgin olive oil, flavored with 4 tablespoons salsa

⅛ avocado

1 medium apple (tennis ball size)

LUNCH

4 ounces beef tenderloin seasoned with your favorite spice blend and grilled

1½ cups steamed green beans

1 medium-size plum

SNACK

2 low-fat string cheese sticks

1 small orange

DINNER

4 ounces Tandoori Chicken (page 237)

6 almonds

1 cup steamed carrots

½ cup cooked spinach

½ cup chopped pineapple

Day 3

BREAKFAST

20/20 LifeStyles High Protein Shake

1 tablespoon nut butter

½ cup cubed melon

LUNCH

4 ounces water-packed tuna mixed with 1 tablespoon low-fat mayonnaise, ½ cup diced celery, and 1 cup sliced carrots

1 medium apple (tennis ball size)

SNACK

2 low-fat string cheese sticks

1 medium apple (tennis ball size)

DINNER

4 ounces Mediterranean Grilled Tuna (page 240)
1½ cups steamed broccoli
1 cup strawberries

Stage 4: Men

1,300–1,700 calories per day

Day 1

BREAKFAST

2 ounces turkey sausage
½ cup low-fat cottage cheese mixed with ¼ cup raspberries, ½ cup blueberries, and 10 walnut halves

SNACK

2 ounces low-sodium sliced turkey breast
½ cup sliced peaches

LUNCH

6 ounces salmon prepared with Mustard-Peppercorn Rub (page 200) and grilled
Steamed-vegetable medley: ½ cup cauliflower, ½ cup broccoli, and ½ cup carrots
1 medium apple (tennis ball size)

SNACK

20/20 LifeStyles Protein Bar

DINNER

6 ounces Roast Chicken (page 231)
Spinach salad: 1½ cups spinach leaves, ½ cup sliced radishes, ½ cup chopped tomatoes, 2 tablespoons dressing of your choice (page 208)
½ cup grapes

Day 2

BREAKFAST

1 cup egg whites scrambled in 1 teaspoon extra-virgin olive oil or canola oil, flavored with 4 tablespoons salsa

1/8 avocado

1 medium apple (tennis ball size)

SNACK

2 ounces low-sodium turkey jerky

½ cup peaches

LUNCH

6 ounces beef tenderloin seasoned with your favorite spice blend and grilled

1½ cups steamed green beans

1 medium-size plum

SNACK

2 low-fat string cheese sticks

1 medium orange (tennis ball size)

DINNER

6 ounces Tandoori Chicken (page 237)

6 almonds

1 cup steamed carrots

½ cup cooked greens such as kale or spinach

½ cup cubed melon

Day 3

BREAKFAST

20/20 LifeStyles High Protein Shake

1 tablespoon nut butter

½ cup peaches or ½ medium banana

SNACK

2 low-fat string cheese sticks

1 cup strawberries

LUNCH

6 ounces water-packed tuna mixed with 1 tablespoon low-fat mayonnaise, ½ cup diced celery, and 1 cup sliced carrots

1 medium-size plum

SNACK

20/20 LifeStyles Protein Bar

DINNER

6 ounces Mediterranean Grilled Tuna (page 240)

1½ cups steamed asparagus

½ cup cubed pineapple

Stage 5: Women

1,100–1,400 calories per day

Day 1

BREAKFAST

1 cup egg whites scrambled in 1 teaspoon extra-virgin olive oil

⅛ avocado

½ cup low-fat strawberry yogurt

LUNCH

4 ounces Avocado Tuna Salad (page 211) served with or on top of 1½ cups spinach, ½ cup chopped tomatoes, ¼ cup sliced mushrooms, ½ cup carrots, 1 tablespoon Simple Lemon Vinaigrette (page 209)

1 medium apple (tennis ball size)

SNACK

2 ounces low-sodium sliced turkey

1 cup berries

DINNER

4 ounces Thai Chicken Satay with Peanut Sauce (page 232)

1½ cups carrots

1 cup nonfat milk

Day 2

BREAKFAST

1 cup egg whites scrambled in 1 teaspoon extra-virgin olive oil, flavored with 4 tablespoons salsa

⅛ avocado

1 medium apple (tennis ball size)

LUNCH

Crustless Smoked Salmon Quiche with Dill (page 246)

1½ cups steamed broccoli

½ cup low-fat strawberry yogurt

SNACK

20/20 LifeStyles Protein Bar

DINNER

4 ounces Curried Chicken Breasts (page 237)

1½ cups Asian Asparagus-and-Orange Salad (page 218)

Day 3

BREAKFAST

20/20 LifeStyles High Protein Shake

1 tablespoon nut butter

½ cup peaches or ½ medium banana

LUNCH

Tuna wrap: 4 ounces water-packed tuna, 1 tablespoon low-fat mayonnaise, and 1–2 lettuce leaves for wrap

1 cup chopped green beans

1 medium-size peach

SNACK

½ cup flavored nonfat Greek yogurt with 2 tablespoons sliced almonds

DINNER

4 ounces Ginger Lime Fish (page 245)

1½ cups steamed asparagus

1 cup strawberries

Stage 5: Men

1,300–1700 calories per day

Day 1

BREAKFAST

1 cup egg whites scrambled in 1 teaspoon extra-virgin olive oil
⅛ avocado
½ cup low-fat strawberry yogurt

SNACK

1 tablespoon nut butter
1 medium apple (tennis ball size)

LUNCH

6 ounces Avocado Tuna Salad (page 211) served with or on top of 1½ cups spinach, ½ cup chopped tomatoes, ¼ cup sliced mushrooms, ½ cup carrots, 1 tablespoon Simple Lemon Vinaigrette (page 209)
1 medium orange (tennis ball size)

SNACK

2 ounces low-sodium sliced turkey
1 cup berries

DINNER

6 ounces Thai Chicken Satay with Peanut Sauce (page 232)
1½ cup carrots
1 cup nonfat milk

Day 2

BREAKFAST

1 cup egg whites scrambled in 1 teaspoon extra-virgin olive oil, flavored with 4 tablespoons salsa
⅛ avocado
1 medium apple (tennis ball size)

SNACK

2 ounces low-sodium turkey jerky

½ cup peaches

LUNCH

Crustless Smoked Salmon Quiche with Dill (page 246)

1½ cups steamed broccoli

1½ cups flavored nonfat yogurt

SNACK

20/20 LifeStyles Protein Bar

DINNER

6 ounces Curried Chicken Breasts (page 237)

1½ cups Asian Asparagus-and-Orange Salad (page 218)

Day 3

BREAKFAST

20/20 LifeStyles High Protein Shake

1 tablespoon nut butter

½ cup peaches or ½ medium banana

SNACK

2 low-fat string cheese sticks

1 cup strawberries

LUNCH

Lettuce wrap burger: 6 ounces very lean ground beef (5% fat), ⅛ avocado, mustard, 1 tablespoon ketchup, 1 tomato slice, 2 large lettuce leaves for wrap

1½ cups green beans

1 medium apple (tennis ball size)

SNACK

½ cup flavored low-fat yogurt with two tablespoons sliced almonds

DINNER

6 ounces Ginger Lime Fish (page 245)

1½ cups steamed broccoli

1 cup strawberries

Stage 6: Women

1,100–1,400 calories per day

Day 1

BREAKFAST

20/20 LifeStyles High Protein Shake
1 tablespoon nut butter
1 medium apple (tennis ball size)

LUNCH

Chicken Caesar salad: 3 ounces grilled chicken breast, 1½ cups romaine lettuce, ½ cup green beans, ½ cup artichoke hearts, 1 tablespoon light Caesar dressing, and ¼ cup (1 ounce) grated Parmesan cheese
½ cup nonfat yogurt

SNACK

¼ cup hummus with 1 cup sliced raw veggies

DINNER

4 ounces Sicilian Tuna Steak (page 242)
Simple salad: 1½ cup salad greens, ½ cup garbanzo beans, and 1 tablespoon of your favorite dressing (page 208)

Day 2

BREAKFAST

2 ounces turkey bacon
Fruity yogurt cup: ½ cup nonfat plain Greek yogurt, ½ cup nonfat blueberry yogurt, 10 walnut halves

LUNCH

4 ounces flank steak prepared with your favorite marinade or rub and grilled, served with or on top of ½ cup garbanzo beans, 1½ cups arugula, ½ cup tomatoes, ½ cup carrots, and 1 tablespoon Red Wine Vinaigrette (page 209)

SNACK

20/20 LifeStyles Protein Bar

DINNER

4 ounces Thai Chicken Satay with Peanut Sauce (page 232)
1½ cups Asian Asparagus-and-Orange Salad (page 218)

Day 3

BREAKFAST

20/20 LifeStyles High Protein Shake
1 tablespoon nut butter
½ cup peaches or ½ medium banana

LUNCH

California Chicken Salad in Lettuce Cups (page 215)
1 cup strawberries

SNACK

½ cup flavored nonfat Greek yogurt with 2 tablespoons sliced almonds

DINNER

4 ounces Herb-Marinated Flank Steak (page 228)
1 cup steamed broccoli
Simple salad: 1½ cup salad greens, ½ cup rinsed garbanzo beans, and 1 tablespoon of your favorite dressing (page 208)

Stage 6: Men

1,300–1700 calories per day

Day 1

BREAKFAST

20/20 LifeStyles High Protein Shake
1 tablespoon nut butter
½ cup cubed pineapple

SNACK

2 tablespoons hummus with ½ cup sliced raw carrots

12 almonds

LUNCH

Chicken Caesar salad: 5 ounces grilled chicken breast, 1½ cups romaine lettuce, ½ cup green beans, ½ cup artichoke hearts, 1 tablespoon light Caesar dressing, and ¼ cup (1 ounce) grated Parmesan cheese

½ cup nonfat yogurt

SNACK

20/20 LifeStyles Protein Bar

DINNER

6 ounces Sicilian Tuna Steak (page 242)

Simple salad: 1½ cups salad greens, ½ cup garbanzo beans, and 1 tablespoon of your favorite dressing (page 208)

Day 2

BREAKFAST

2 ounces turkey bacon

Fruity yogurt cup: ½ cup nonfat plain Greek yogurt, ½ cup nonfat blueberry yogurt, and 10 walnut halves

SNACK

2 ounces low-sodium turkey jerky

½ cup peaches

LUNCH

6 ounces flank steak prepared with your favorite marinade or rub and grilled, served with or on top of ½ cup garbanzo beans, 1½ cups arugula, ½ cup tomatoes, ½ cup carrots, and 1 tablespoon Red Wine Vinaigrette (page 209)

SNACK

20/20 LifeStyles Protein Bar

DINNER

6 ounces Thai Chicken Satay with Peanut Sauce (page 232)

1½ cups Asian Asparagus-and-Orange Salad (page 218)

Day 3

BREAKFAST

20/20 LifeStyles High Protein Shake
1 tablespoon nut butter
½ cup peaches or ½ medium banana

SNACK

2 low-fat string cheese sticks
1 medium apple (tennis ball size)

LUNCH

6 ounces California Chicken Salad in Lettuce Cups (page 215)
1 cup strawberries

SNACK

½ cup flavored low-fat yogurt with 2 tablespoons sliced almonds

DINNER

6 ounces Herb-Marinated Flank Steak (page 228)
1½ cups steamed carrots
Simple salad: 1½ cups salad greens, ½ cup rinsed garbanzo beans, 1 tablespoon of your favorite salad dressing (page 208)

Stage 7: Women

1,100–1,400 calories per day

Day 1

BREAKFAST

¾ cup egg whites scrambled with ¼ cup (1 ounce) grated low-fat Cheddar cheese, ½ cup black beans, ¼ avocado, and 1 tablespoon salsa

LUNCH

Toasted Quinoa, Chicken, and Avocado Salad (page 224)
½ cup sliced raw veggies

SNACK

¼ cup hummus with 1 cup sliced raw veggies

DINNER

4 ounces pork tenderloin marinated in Latin Marinade (page 194) and roasted

1½ cups steamed broccoli

1 cup blueberries

Day 2

BREAKFAST

Cinnamon oats: ½ cup steel-cut oats cooked in water, 5 chopped walnut halves, and a dash or more of cinnamon

1 cup egg whites scrambled in 1 teaspoon extra-virgin olive oil

LUNCH

4 ounces Curried Chicken Breasts (page 237)

1½ cups salad greens with ½ cup garbanzo beans, topped with 1 tablespoon dressing

SNACK

20/20 LifeStyles Protein Bar

DINNER

4 ounces Slow Cooker White Bean Chicken Chili (page 226)

1½ cups asparagus

Day 3

BREAKFAST

20/20 LifeStyles High Protein Shake

1 tablespoon nut butter

½ banana

LUNCH

4 ounces salmon marinated in your marinade of choice (page 194) and grilled

1½ cups steamed green beans

1 cup strawberries

SNACK

½ cup flavored nonfat Greek yogurt with 2 tablespoons sliced almonds

DINNER

4 ounces flank steak or beef tenderloin prepared with Coffee Rub (page 199) and grilled

½ cup brown rice

1½ cups steamed zucchini

Stage 7: Men

1,300–1,700 calories per day

Day 1

BREAKFAST

¾ cup egg whites scrambled with ¼ cup (1 ounce) grated low-fat Cheddar cheese, ½ cup black beans, ¼ avocado, and 1 tablespoon salsa

SNACK

2 tablespoons hummus with ½ cup sliced raw carrots

12 almonds

LUNCH

Toasted Quinoa, Chicken, and Avocado Salad (page 224)

½ cup sliced raw veggies

SNACK

20/20 LifeStyles Protein Bar

DINNER

6 ounces pork tenderloin marinated in Latin Marinade (page 194) and roasted

1½ cups steamed broccoli

½ cup nonfat yogurt

Day 2

BREAKFAST

Cinnamon oats: ½ cup steel-cut oats cooked in water, 5 chopped walnut halves, and a dash or more of cinnamon

1 cup egg whites scrambled in 1 teaspoon extra-virgin olive oil

SNACK

2 hard-boiled eggs

1 medium apple (tennis ball size)

LUNCH

6 ounces Curried Chicken Breasts (page 237)

1 cup romaine lettuce, ½ cup chopped tomatoes, ½ cup garbanzo beans, and 1 tablespoon Red Wine Vinaigrette (page 209)

SNACK

20/20 LifeStyles Protein Bar

DINNER

4 ounces Slow Cooker White Bean Chicken Chili (page 226)

1½ cups asparagus

Day 3

BREAKFAST

20/20 LifeStyles High Protein Shake

1 tablespoon nut butter

1 cup blueberries

SNACK

2 low-fat string cheese sticks

1 medium apple (tennis ball size)

LUNCH

6 ounces salmon marinated in your marinade of choice (page 194) and grilled

1½ cups steamed green beans

1 cup strawberries

SNACK

½ cup flavored low-fat yogurt with 2 tablespoons sliced almonds

DINNER

6 ounces flank steak or beef tenderloin prepared with Coffee Rub (page 199) and grilled

½ cup brown rice

1½ cups steamed zucchini

Further Reading and Online Resources

20/20 LIFESTYLES CLINIC

Since the Love Diet and 20/20 LifeStyles are based on the same principles, you can connect with our team of experts at the clinic if you need additional assistance with the plan. We have physicians, registered dietitians, personal trainers, and licensed counselors on staff who can address specific questions or offer guidance on areas that may be challenging to you.

20/20 LifeStyles
4455 148th Avenue Northeast
Bellevue, WA 98007
425.861.6258 or 877.559.2020
www.2020lifestyles.com

CODEPENDENT RESOURCES

Codependent No More, by Melody Beattie
Codependent No More Workbook, also by Melody Beattie

EXTENDED SUPPLEMENT SECTION

Here's a list of additional supplements, beyond the three recommended in the supplement section on page 91, and how they've been shown to benefit health. Consult with your personal doctor before taking any of the following supplements:

Vitamins

Folic acid: Most of us have heard about folic acid deficiencies related to birth defects, but folic acid does much more than prevent spina bifida in newborns. This important B vitamin can help regulate homocysteine, an amino acid found in the blood, which at high levels can cause hardening of the arteries and dementia. Daily dosage: 300 mcg.

Vitamin C: A powerful antioxidant, vitamin C is related to lower risk of cataract formation and is preventative against hardening of the arteries. Vitamin C is water soluble, which means any amount taken in excess of what your body needs will be eliminated. Daily dosage: 200 mg.

Beta carotene: Beta carotene is converted to vitamin A within the body, where it is then used to help with vision issues, assist the immune system, and promote healthy skin, hair, bones, teeth, and nails. Taking vitamin A directly can cause toxicity, but that does not occur with beta carotene. Because beta carotene is fat soluble, you'll want to make sure you don't take too much. Daily dosage: 2,000 IU.

Vitamins B_6 and B_{12}: B_6 and B_{12} can help keep your arteries pliable, protect against nerve damage, and improve the circulation of oxygen throughout the body. Daily dosage: 20 mg of B_6 and 1,200 mcg of B_{12}.

Coenzyme Q_{10} (CoQ_{10}): CoQ_{10} is an antioxidant made in the body that is also available in supplement form. CoQ_{10} can improve muscle and tissue health, benefitting your entire body, including your heart, skin, and gums. Daily dosage: 100 mg.

Alpha-lipoic acid: Also known as ALA, alpha-lipoic acid is critical for energy production at the cellular level and is also an important antioxidant that can help neutralize the effects of damaging free radicals. ALA also helps activate insulin receptors, which will help prevent insulin resistance. Daily dosage: 50 mg.

Minerals

Calcium: The average American only gets 60 to 80 percent of their required daily amount of calcium. If you exercise, you lose more calcium in your perspiration, making supplementation even more important. It's important to note that since calcium and iron are absorbed in the same pathway, they should not be taken at the same time of day. Daily dosage: 600 mg.

Iron: You need sufficient iron in your body to help maintain a healthy number of red blood cells, which are responsible for carrying oxygen to all your cells. Daily dosage: premenopausal women: 10 mg; men and postmenopausal women: no iron supplementation needed.

Zinc: Zinc helps with fat burning, assists with the building of protein and muscle, enables the production of a pigment important to eye health, and strengthens your immune and nervous systems. Zinc is also lost through sweating so it's important to consider if you exercise often. Daily dose: 11 mg.

Magnesium: Magnesium is necessary for proper heart function, effectiveness of the body's insulin, and healthy bones and teeth. Daily dose: 200 mg.

THE LOVE DIET GUIDE TO BETTER SLEEP AND LESS STRESS

While making changes to your diet and getting enough exercise are essential to successful weight loss, they're not the only factors important to creating a permanent transformation. How much sleep you get and the quality of your shut-eye as well as the level of stress you endure each day and your tools for managing it can have a significant impact on your weight too. Both stress and sleep can affect appetite, energy, metabolism, and most certainly overall well-being.

In this guide, we'll share ways that you can improve your stress-management skills and sleep habits. Let's take a look at these important lifestyle factors.

The Stress-Weight Connection

You're not imagining things when you feel as though stress creates aches and pains, disrupts your mood, or changes your habits around food. When you endure physical stress, emotional stress, anxiety, or depression, there are chemical changes that occur in the body that have very real and noticeable ramifications. A cascade of hormones is fired off in response, which increases heart rate, blood pressure, and breathing rate and tightens your muscles. Your body was designed to respond this way—but only in desperate, life-or-death situations.

The chemical changes that occur in your body as a response to stress are part of what's called your fight-or-flight response. In our hunter-gatherer ancestors, these chemicals were triggered to help increase the chance of survival in a crisis situation. The adrenal gland, a small gland located on top of the kidney, would secrete norepinephrine and epinephrine to make you more agile and heighten your awareness, and cortisol would help maintain functions if you were injured.

Many of us wouldn't be here if it weren't for our built-in stress response—it likely saved many lives, helping our ancestors evade things like a charging saber-toothed tiger or endure times of famine.

Fast-forward thousands of years and these very same stress hormones that used to help people stay alive have now begun to harm us. That's because they're designed as a response to acute stress—fleeting moments of extreme demand in the face of a threat—and not chronic stress, which is when you are repeatedly exposed to stressful situations.

Chronic stress is a long-term event. It can be caused by physical illness or injury, but usually it's a result of everyday problems related to money, work, family, relationships—pressures from which there is no break (some days make running from a tiger seem not so bad). This constant exposure to stress leads to a steady production of stress hormones, such as insulin and steroids, which increase levels of inflammation chemicals and negatively affect metabolism, energy, mood, immune health, and food cravings. Chronic stress also triggers an ancient response that allows your body to seek and store extra calories in the form of fat.

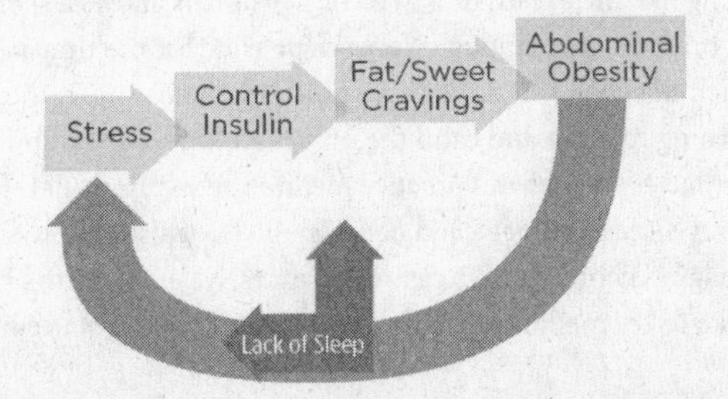

The stress hormone we're most concerned about is cortisol, which you've probably heard is bad, but you might not be aware of how severely it can impact your health and weight issues. Excess cortisol puts you on the fast track to insulin resistance, which will promote greater fat storage in your cells and weight gain in the abdominal region. As your belly fat accumulates, so too does your risk for developing the type of serious metabolic imbalance that is the precursor to type 2 diabetes. Cortisol can also increase hunger and drive you toward fatty and sugary foods (see chart; lack of sleep doesn't help either, which we'll discuss in the next section).

How can you tell if you're managing stress well? You look to your waist size. Your increasing belly fat and waist size are indicators of how well you are managing stress in your life—stress increases belly fat! And stress is contagious.

To minimize cortisol production, you have to look to what triggers it in the first place—stress. While you may not be able to remove stress from your life, you can practice techniques that restore calm and quell the secretion of stress hormones. Here are a few stress-busting methods we recommend:

Exercise to beat stress: Exercise is one of the most powerful fighters of stress and its negative effects (remember: it's a magic potion!). Aerobic exercise in particular has the distinct ability to both energize and calm, helping balance moods by easing anxiety and depression, and buffering the effects of stress. Exercise lowers the body's levels of stress hormones, especially adrenaline and cortisol. Even just a short walk can help put the brakes on your body's stress response.

Meditate to cool cortisol production: Learning to the quiet the mind is a powerful way to cut off the body's stress response before it even begins. If you can learn to operate from a calm mind, you can take the power out of the stress response by changing your initial reaction: "Oh, that's not a tiger! It's just a bill I have to pay on time—I'll put it on the calendar." The incredible thing is that a more measured response in your mind will ultimately benefit your body by cutting off the production of those inflammatory, weight-promoting hormones.

Meditation is a way of training the mind to obtain a singular focus, whether it's on something like the breath or a mantra. This focus allows a state of peace to settle in the brain as other thoughts are swept aside for the time being. It is an exercise in which the goal is to do nothing other than quiet the mind. Research shows that learning to quiet and calm the mind can have a profound impact on the body and mind—people who practice meditation regularly develop less hypertension, heart disease, anxiety, and depression. They also find it easier to give up health-damaging habits such as cigarettes, excessive alcohol, and binge eating.

If you'd like to try meditation, here a few tips for getting started:

Start small: Begin by dedicating at least five minutes in the morning each day to focusing on your breath and quieting your mind. Increase the time as you begin to feel comfortable with the quietness.

Download a meditation app or use a timer: There are several free meditation apps available such as Calm and Headspace. These will provide a short, guided meditation and give you a seven-day entry-level plan. If downloading an app seems like too much trouble, just set a timer so you're not constantly checking the time to see if you're done.

Get comfortable: Settle yourself in a comfortable chair or on the floor with pillows to prop you up. There's no one right way to meditate; just be sure you won't be disturbed and you are in a position that allows good posture, which will allow for increased oxygen and airflow throughout the body.

Be patient: You won't feel the benefits in the first three minutes of meditation, but once you begin to create a consistent habit, you'll find you actually crave the peaceful pause. And don't be afraid of making adjustments—if you don't find that morning is working for you, try an evening meditation or look for a new space in your home to try.

In addition to meditation, increasing your positive self-talk and self-love can strengthen your stress tolerance. When you focus on positive thoughts, feel-good hormones such as serotonin are produced, helping you feel calm and in control.

Incorporating these techniques for better stress management will help improve your quality of life, lifting you from a state of despair to a state of capable calm: *I can do this*. Of course, they will also help put an end to the increased fat storage and metabolic disturbances caused by excess cortisol; with these factors removed, steady weight loss will be much easier to achieve.

Let's look at one other important part of your life that can help increase your success with the Love Diet: sleep. The bonus is that better sleep will also make you more equipped to deal with stress. It's a win-win!

Better Sleep: The Other Key to Controlling Cravings and Losing Weight

We spend one third of lives sleeping—at least we used to. In decades past, the average amount of sleep per night was eight to nine hours, but now we're lucky if we're getting seven. Getting less sleep doesn't just make you tired; it can also lead to a decline in mental performance, weight gain, cravings for high-fat and high-sugar foods, insulin resistance, increased levels of inflammatory proteins and cortisol, elevated blood pressure, and more. The Centers for Disease Control and Prevention has even gone so far as to call insufficient sleep a "public health epidemic," citing its link to increased incidence of car accidents and on-the-job disasters.

The question is: why aren't we getting enough sleep? There are numerous reasons. We're working longer hours and more night shifts, taking on more activi-

FEWER ZZZs EQUALS LOWER CALORIC BURN

Your body burns calories naturally throughout the day through a process called non-exercise activity thermogenesis, or NEAT. Thermogenesis is defined as heat production, and it's the process by which we burn calories in our bodies. Many things contribute to your NEAT—how much you fidget, how much you slouch or sit up straight, or even how often you use your hands while talking. Sleep deprivation can dramatically *lower* your daily NEAT, without you even noticing it. So you have two choices: you can either become a jittery, fidgety, gesticulating live wire to burn extra calories or you can simply work on improving your sleep. We vote for option number two!

ties and commitments (for our kids and ourselves), playing video games, watching TV, and surfing the Internet . . . all the while drinking caffeinated beverages throughout the day that prevent us from falling asleep easily at night.

Modern society's increase in obesity has contributed too. Being overweight or obese increases your risk for sleep-disrupting conditions such as sleep apnea, snoring, and restless legs syndrome. But it may be the lack of sleep that perpetuates weight gain in the first place.

Have you noticed that you eat more when you're sleep deprived? It's not a coincidence. Poor sleep leads to less production of leptin, which you may recall is an important appetite-shutoff hormone. When leptin is released from your cells, it sends the "I'm full" signal and you know it's time to stop eating. When it's not released, it's all too easy to continue plowing through calories even though you've already had enough.

Less shut-eye also increases the production of ghrelin (think of it as growlin'—because that's what it makes your stomach do), which tells your body it's in need of food. The nudges for food can be strong and constant, programming you to search for quickly satisfying foods, specifically those that are high in calories and carbohydrates.

The combination of less leptin and more ghrelin caused by sleep deprivation is a disastrous one when it comes to your diet, leading to as many as 500 more calories eaten per day. Over time, these excess calories will inevitably result in consistent and significant weight gain. The good news is that improving your sleep habits can go a long way toward shutting off the cycle of appetite dysfunction.

While many of the strategies for better sleep require some effort, paying your sleep some attention is the first priority. How many hours of solid sleep are you getting each night? When you consider your typical evening, can you see behaviors that might be contributing to lost sleep? Are you eating and drinking late at night? Staring at a screen up until the moment you close your eyes? Drinking coffee or caffeinated soda late in the afternoon? These can all create sleep disturbances. Let's look at several proven ways to improve both the quality and duration of your sleep:

Exercise five days per week in the morning or afternoon: Aerobic exercise promotes restfulness, but it can also leave you feeling too alert for sleep if you work out too late in the day.

Establish a bedtime routine: While you might think watching TV or scrolling through webpages helps you wind down, it actually can delay the production of melatonin, the hormone that promotes sleep. Instead, try going for an evening walk, taking a bath, performing easy stretches, or reading some fiction. Aim to start one of these calming activities forty-five minutes before you go to bed.

Create a better sleeping space: A cool and dark bedroom is best. Keep your room temperature between 65 and 68 degrees, and consider blackout shades if your room tends to be somewhat bright at night due to neighboring lights or night owls in the other room. Complete darkness will help trigger melatonin.

Watch your diet and drinks—and the clock: Avoiding spicy foods and alcohol at least three to four hours before bed can minimize disturbances caused by both—spicy foods can wage acid reflux revenge, and alcohol will prevent you from falling into the deepest, most restorative levels of sleep. Coffee consumption should be shutdown at least six hours before bedtime.

Get the kids and pets out of your bed: A good night's sleep is impossible to get when little ones are squirming and flailing about, especially when you're all squished together. Plus, sleeping in their own bed will be better for them too—they need ten to twelve hours of sleep a night to your seven to eight.

Acknowledgments

During the course of our lives, we are blessed when special individuals enrich our endeavors to ultimately improve our lives. I have been fortunate to have an amazing group of mentors, supporters, and key influencers over the course of my life. This is the type of book that results from years of experience, working with gifted professionals and taking the opportunity to reflect on the outcomes of patient successes and failures. Many thanks and much gratitude are due to the individuals who made this book a reality. Their remarkable talents are the foundation of *The Love Diet.*

Mark Dedomenico, M.D., coauthor and medical director of the 20/20 LifeStyles Clinic, is a visionary physician whose medical career made this book possible. I thank him for believing in me and sharing the principles of his clinic for *The Love Diet.* His sincere dedication to his patients is the premise of *The Love Diet,* ultimately making it like no other "diet book." Along with my father, Bruno Peraglie, M.D., they both share an integrity and value in treating the "whole" person, where love and self-respect are at the core of individual success for better health.

Thank you to the entire 20/20 LifeStyles Clinic team: Barry Wolborsky, Ph.D., for the endless review and coordination of information; Rainer Rey, for his creative interpretation of the clinic success and informative content, as well as the in-depth narrative recollections of our patient stories; registered dietitians Andy Miller, M.S., R.D., and Amanda Gonsalves-Wood, R.D., for their nutritional insight and detailed menus; and Judy Crane, Jen Masterson, and Linda Rackner for their administrative organization.

Thank you to the *Love Diet* team at HarperOne: Gideon Weil, Amy Van Langen, Suzanne Wickham, and Lisa Zuniga. Your partnership has been amazing in this journey. A special thank you to Gideon Weil, whose inspiration and support is only part of the extraordinary vision he has for this book. To Gretchen Lees, thank you for sharing your excitement and creative views for this book. The engaging language and organization of the information owe much to your hard work and attention to detail.

Thank you to my friend and agent, Heidi Krupp. Everything is possible with your talents and vision. Your ideas set the course for an amazing future.

To the special individuals who shared their words of wisdom through personal stories in this book, may your insight and experiences bring health and happiness to those who seek a healthier way of living.

Finally, to Shawn, my husband, and our children, Gigi and William: without your support and inspiration, this project would not have been possible. The love and respect that stem from family are the foundation of health, success, and happiness.

Index

About the Authors

CONNIE GUTTERSEN, R.D., Ph.D., is the *New York Times* bestselling author of *The Sonoma Diet,* a registered dietitian and nutrition instructor at the world-famous Culinary Institute of America, and has consulted with a broad range of corporations and Fortune 500 companies. She lives with her family in Northern California.

MARK DEDOMENICO, M.D., is the founder and medical director of the renowned 20/20 Lifestyles program. A former cardiovascular surgeon, he has done extensive research in the field of metabolic disease control and weight management to correct metabolic disorders without medication. He lives in Seattle, Washington.